YOUR PAINFUL

YOUR PAINFUL NECK AND BACK

A complete guide to self-help

HOW TO TREAT YOURSELF
WHEN TO GET HELP
WHAT HELP TO GET

Dr James W. Fisk, MD, DCH, MRCGP

Illustrations by Isla Trapski

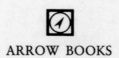

ARROW BOOKS

Arrow Books Limited
62–65 Chandos Place, London WC2N 4NW

An imprint of Century Hutchinson Limited

London Melbourne Sydney Auckland Johannesburg
and agencies throughout the world

First published 1987

Phototypeset in Linotron Sabon, 10 on 11½ point by
Input Typesetting Limited, London SW19 8DR
Printed and bound in Great Britain by
The Guernsey Press Co. Ltd., Guernsey Channel Islands

ISBN 0 09 952000 1

Contents

Preface

This book is dedicated to Ivan Illich, whose writings have stimulated radical thinking both within and outside the medical profession. He has been a prime mover in the patient self help movement. At times, in order to make his point, he goes a bit too far, but this should not detract from the value of his work.

The ability to help oneself is important, and adds to human dignity, but to do it intelligently requires knowledge. This is the hard bit, but to take more responsibility for our own health without knowledge is asking for trouble.

It is the intent of this book to supply the necessary knowledge about one part of our anatomy, the spine, in a manner which is understandable to the non-professional reader.

The basic information takes up a lot of space, for which I apologize, but there are no short cuts to learning what should be known in order to look after your own sore neck or back. I suggest the reader who just wishes to be told what or what not to do should go straight to the section on treatment (section 4, pages 107–58).

I have tried to exclude personal opinions disguised as 'facts'. This has not always been possible: there is insufficient scientific information in all instances.

I have been accused of not sufficiently emphasising the dangers of self help. (This accusation is a favourite ploy of vested interests.) It would be easy to frighten the reader with horror stories about what might happen if the correct professional advice is not immediately obtained, but I have resisted the temptation to do this, and instead I have added a short section at the end of the book which lists the possible hazards.

Hazard is an integral part of our existence, it adds spice to life. Rarely, it may even be hazardous going to the doctor, physiotherapist, or chiropractor.

I hope that this book will encourage the reader to take a more active personal role when having to cope with this all too common problem. It will not affect the quantity of life but may certainly affect the quality. One can ask for little more.

Introduction

It has been said humanity can be divided into three groups: those who make things happen; those who watch things happening; and those who wonder what in heaven is happening.

To suffer a sore neck or back gives one the doubtful distinction of belonging to the third group.

Attempts to rectify this situation have been made. I have in front of me seven books for the general reader on back pain – how to treat your own backache, what causes it, what to do to prevent it – and this is only a small sample of what is available on the market. These books are written by experts and yet the advice given to the sufferer varies considerably; sometimes, indeed, what is said in one book totally contradicts what is said in another. This diversity of advice is similar to the dilemma faced by the overweight: bookshops have rows of books on various diets for losing weight.

There is an old truism in medical circles: if there are many cures there is no cure. This is so with back and neck pain. In the majority of instances there is no disease to cure. What we are really having to cope with is an ageing process that has become painful for one reason or another. The best we can expect is relief from the pain, and this can be achieved in several different ways.

So why another book to add to the confusion?

A good question.

That such confusion exists calls for an attempt to clear away the fog. It is time we learnt to help ourselves more than we have in the past, but to do so requires knowledge. To make any intelligent decision requires access to all available knowledge – information about what is known and unknown.

So, this book sets out to provide information not generally

available elsewhere in a way that is understandable to the general reader. This information is based on many years' work in research into back problems and many years of looking after thousands of neck and back pain sufferers.

Those unfortunate enough to suffer a sore neck or back will not be short of advice from friends and relatives: 'Go to so and so! (S)he fixed my back.' So and so may be a GP who 'tweaks' backs, an orthopaedic surgeon, a physical medicine specialist, a chiropractor, a physiotherapist, an osteopath, or a naturopath. That there is such a diversity of experts available should give food for thought – the commercial viability of looking after humanity's sore necks and backs must be at least partly responsible. This book aims to guide the reader through the maze of alternatives: when to go it alone; when to get help and from whom; how to assess any advice and treatment given.

Obviously, those who read this book will have or have had trouble with their necks and backs. Back and neck pain bedevils most of us at some stage in life, whatever our sex and whatever we do. The sedentary worker is no less prone to it than the manual worker. Women have just as much trouble with their spines as men. In fact, women tend to get more trouble with their necks than men. Perhaps social custom has something to do with this: it is not considered ladylike to stick the posterior up in the air when bending, and the ladylike bend puts more stress on the neck. Or possibly we males are the real pain in women's necks.

It has been estimated that at least eighty per cent of us will suffer a debilitating attack of low back pain at some stage of our lives, and it has been estimated that back problems cost industrialized nations literally billions of pounds every year.

Why is humankind prone to so much trouble from the spine? It has been argued humanity has paid a high price for having the temerity to stand on two feet: evolution has not caught up with the stresses imposed by the upright stance. Yet engineers tell us that for standing on two feet the human spine could not be bettered. Our early ancestors were hunters and could not have survived with weak backs. Nature had adequate time to weed out those with defective spines.

It has also been suggested that having successfully got on to two feet the effort has been such that we have had to sit down and rest, and have been doing too much sitting ever since. One scientist studied back problems amongst native populations in India and found them to be virtually non-existent. He concluded this was because they did not sit in modern easy chairs: they squatted or sat cross-legged on the floor with their backs bent forward. Because of this, their backs were comfortable in the bent-forward position and were not strained during everyday bending activities. This sounds feasible but there are possible flaws in the argument. I read somewhere that the audience at strip-club shows consists mainly of elderly bald-headed men. This does not necessarily mean your hair will fall out if you watch ladies undressing on the stage. So too, the fact that you sit with your back bent forwards is not necessarily the cause of your freedom from spinal pain.

More recent research also points to prolonged sitting as being a key factor in the early breakdown of our spines. We will return to this problem later.

It has been argued that back and neck pain is a comparatively modern epidemic: a by-product of the existence humankind now has to cope with. It has been calculated the average person only uses about ten per cent of the energy that was expended in daily living fifty years ago. Thus we may be suffering from the ease of modern transport, labour-saving devices, lifts, easy chairs, and so on. In other words, from the lack of daily exercise. Fortunately for our forebears statisticians were not so evident in days long past so we have no figures to compare the relative frequency of back problems then and now. But it certainly seems that back and neck problems are more prevalent than just a few years ago.

Another important factor to be considered is the effect of emotional stresses imposed on us in this day and age. Stress of this sort can lead to tightness in our muscles, particularly those in the neck and back. It is no coincidence that people and things can give us pain at the two extremes of the spine: in the neck and butt.

To understand the possible causes of neck and back pain and

what to do about it requires some basic knowledge about how the spine is structured, how it functions, and how things may go wrong. This will be covered in the first few chapters. The next section aims to show you how to manage your own neck and back pain, when *not* to go it alone, who to go to for help, and how to evaluate such help.

For some time people have felt that society has become too dependent on the medical profession: we have become over-medicalized. Dependency to such an extent is demoralizing and has led to an instinctive revolt, hence the blossoming of alternative medicine cults. This is just jumping out of the frying pan into the fire.

The recent explosion of scientific knowledge has widened the gap between the knows and don't knows, partly because scientific discussion is conducted in jargon incomprehensible to the average reader. This explosion of scientific knowledge has led to increasing specialization and fragmentation within the medical profession too, for no single mind can encompass more than what is known about one small segment of the whole. This specialization has its own built-in dangers: the specialist gets to know more and more about less and less until he knows everything about very little. He also becomes increasingly ignorant about other branches of medicine until he is incapable of forming any judgement on the role and importance of his own sphere within the context of other human knowledge.

In the midst of such proliferating knowledge I feel it is now up to the individual to make the effort to understand more about his or her own body. To do this, information in a comprehensible form is needed. Sore necks and backs are not killers but they do account for a considerable proportion of human misery. I hope that this book will help you to understand this one small field of medicine and thus help you to regain some independence and insight.

Evolution in a Nutshell: the Development of the Spine

Animal and plant life first started in the sea: there was no land available at that time. Plants were able to build up organic compounds from simple elements obtained in their immediate surroundings, so they got stuck in one spot. Animals depended on organic nutrition so they had to move around to find it. Those primitive forms of life that could move the fastest had a better chance of survival, and a torpedo or cigar shape is most effective for moving quickly through water. Muscles were needed for fast movement. The muscles need something rigid to be attached to, so a primitive spine evolved. Originally this was a hollow tube filled by a jelly-like substance, strong enough to brace the side-to-side movement of the fish. Paddles or fins were needed to improve mobility. With increasing size and complexity a more rigid structure was required to withstand increased compression forces, so a stronger spine developed. This was first made of cartilage and then of bone. Bone is too rigid so it had to be jointed, thus segments of cartilage were retained as these joints.

Getting on to terra firma created problems. To get the body off the ground required strengthening of the fins, so they became more fleshy and developed internal bone structure. At the rear end this bone structure became attached to the spine, to help transmit the body weight. The front fins became detached from the head so they could both move independently.

To start with, both the spine and the hind fins/limbs took part in locomotion. As the hind limbs became more efficient they completely took over the function of locomotion. The spine was relieved of this job and it became less flexible and shorter, but also stronger.

Getting up on two feet also created problems. Our ancestors were tree-shrew-like animals, using four-footed locomotion. As they evolved from animals which ran along branches to animals which grasped branches their torsos became shorter and their limbs longer. Those that got down on the ground to seek food elsewhere, the survivors at times of food shortage, developed longer hind limbs. They evolved from using four legs for movement becoming occasionally two legged, and, eventually, habitually two legged.

To stand at ease on two legs required several adjustments. The pelvic bones, those attaching the hips to the low spine, had to shorten and flare out in order to provide a firm floor and support for the stomach contents and also a wider base for the legs to improve ease of balance. The hips and knees had to straighten out. The hips and pelvis did not straighten out completely so the spine had to do the rest of the straightening.

The spine is divided into three sections (see Fig. 1): the neck (cervical) spine consisting of seven separate blocks of bone (vertebrae): the chest (thoracic) spine with twelve separate blocks of bone and ribs attached to each separate block; and the low back (lumbar) spine with five separate blocks. Because the chest part of the spine was more or less fixed by the attached rib cage this straightening up of the spine had to happen in the low back (lumbar) spine. This created a reverse curve in this region. To further balance the counter curve the neck also had to bend backwards. Having these two reverse curves made it possible to stand upright with a balanced stance, without a tendency to fall flat on our faces or flat on our backs, and with our eyes looking straight ahead.

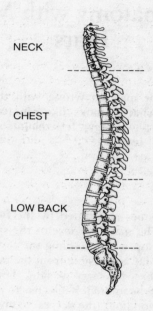

NECK

CHEST

LOW BACK

Figure 1 *The human spine:* The further down the spine the larger the blocks of bone: they have to carry an increasing weight load. Note the backward curve of the neck and low back. When man started to walk on two feet the hips did not completely straighten out, so the spine has to take off at an angle to the vertical — hence the need for a reverse curve in the low back. The main curve in the chest part of the spine is held by the attachments of the rib cage. In order to see straight forward and to stop falling flat on our faces it has been necessary for the neck to bend backwards. Such a shape is ideal for absorbing compression shocks. If the spine was straight up and down any compression stress would be transmitted straight down to the low back. The curves allow such loads to be spread sideways, thus reducing the load on the low back.

SECTION 1
Structure and Function of the Spine: Anatomy with Minimal Tears

To understand what may go wrong with the spine requires knowledge about what it looks like (anatomy) and how it normally functions (physiology). It is the intention to make this a painless process of learning!

Bones

The shape of the bones is dictated by the function they were designed to fulfil. The main purpose of the spine is to provide a stable framework on which to hang the rest of the body and to keep the head as far as possible from the tail. Because of our upright stance it has to carry weight. Some movement is necessary so it has to be jointed. It also has to provide protection for the communication lines (the nerves) to and from the central control (the brain) to the rest of the body. This requires a bony canal with openings at each side for the entry and exit of nerves joining the main trunk line.

The spine consists of twenty-four blocks of bone (vertebrae), seven in the neck, twelve in the chest part of the spine with attached ribs, and five in the low back. These blocks get gradually larger down the spine – they have to carry more weight. If the blocks of bone were piled on top of each other they would form a straight pile. Our curves, attractive or otherwise, are due to the shape of the joints between each block, the discs.

Looked at from above, these blocks of bone are roughly oval in shape (see Fig. 2), becoming slightly kidney shaped in the low

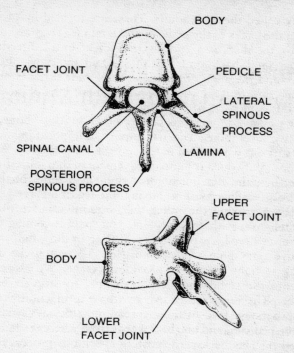

Figure 2 *Top and side view of a typical vertebra:* Note the solid weight-bearing body, the rim of bone protecting the canal which contains the main nerve trunk, and the side arms which provide attachments and leverage for muscles.

back. From both sides of the back of the block of bone (the body of the vertebra) project two arms (pedicles). These form the sides of the canal for the main nerve trunk. These pedicles are joined to each other by a further two plates of bone (laminae) forming the back wall of the nerve trunk canal.

So far we have each block of bone (the body of the vertebra) separated from the next by a joint, the disc, and behind that a bony canal to protect the main nerve trunk. If the disc was the only joint we would tend to wobble about in all directions. To stabilize the spine and to limit directions of movement to those suitable to our requirements there are a further two joints, commonly called the facet joints. These are formed by projections from the backs of the pedicles and laminae. The movement allowed by the discs is a rocking movement in all directions. These other small back joints mainly slide up and down against each other and the angles or planes of the joint surfaces determine which direction movement can or cannot take place. This varies in different parts of the spine.

So now we have three joints between each block of bone, the disc and two facet joints. This has important implications when trying to sort out where pain in the spine is coming from. When examining a joint which is injured movement of that joint should aggravate the pain. But imagine the spine as a series of three-legged stools (see Fig. 3). Try moving one leg of a three-legged stool without moving the other two. So you can see that if someone tells you with certainty that your pain is coming from a disc or elsewhere he is probably whistling in the wind.

To move our spine requires muscles. These muscles need something to hang on to, to provide leverage. We also need attachments for stabilizing ties, ligaments, to stop excessive movement. These are provided by three projections called spinous processes. Two of these spread out sideways from the back of the pedicles, and one backwards from where the laminae join together. This backward (posterior) spinous process is the

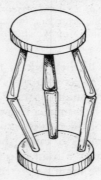

Figure 3 It is impossible to move one leg of a three-legged stool without some movement in the other two.

only part of the spine which can be felt from the outside. When standing upright the tips of these spines can be felt as a more or less vertical line. Very few of us are put together perfectly and sometimes one of these spines is not quite in line with the next, but this does not mean that the underlying back joints are out of line. Anyone telling you this is also whistling in the wind.

Thus we have the structure of a unit of the spine fulfilling all that is required: stability, ability to carry weight, and protection for the main nerve trunk.

The discs

These are the main joints between the blocks of bone, the body of each vertebra. They have to cope with constant pressure, they have to absorb shocks, compression and twisting stresses, and also have to allow limited movement. To carry out these functions requires characteristics unlike other joints. Since the 1930s when it was discovered that these discs sometimes ruptured and caused severe back and leg pain, they have been the subject of a vast amount of research, and we now know quite a lot about how they are constructed (see Fig. 4).

In essence, each disc consists of a semi-fluid centre, the nucleus, surrounded by semi-elastic rings of cartilage, the

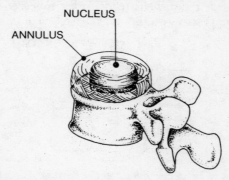

Figure 4 *The Disc:* Each disc is attached to the vertebra by a ring of cartilage.

annulus. These rings of cartilage consist of collagen fibres. Collagen is the tough substance that ties all our tissues together. It has the ability to return to its original length after any sudden stretch, though if it is subject to severe stretch it may remain deformed. It also has a quality known as *visco-elasticity*: even a moderate stretch if maintained for too long will lead to the loss of ability to return fully to its original length after the stretch has stopped.

The rings of cartilage are arranged so that the fibres of the collagen of each ring run in a different direction from those of the next ring, something like the coats of an onion. This means that in whatever direction the back is twisted some of the rings will be able to oppose the twist directly.

Each ring is attached to a plate of cartilage, the end plate, which covers the top and bottom surface of each vertebra. The fibres of the rings along the back wall of the disc are not so well arranged, they tend just to run up and down. This is a potential weak spot where the rings may give way if overstressed.

The semi-fluid centre of the disc (the nucleus) allows any compression load on the spine to be spread in all directions (see Fig. 5). Any impact stress is thus dissipated. It also allows a rocking movement when the spine is bent: the vertebra above literally rolls over the nucleus, like a plank over a barrel, when the back is bent (see Fig. 6). It also means that when the spine is bent forwards the nucleus tends to get squeezed backwards, putting the most stress on the weaker back wall of the annulus.

COMPRESSION LOAD

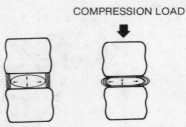

Figure 5 *Spread of compression load within the disc:* The semi-fluid nucleus ensures that any compression loading is dispersed in all directions inside the disc, thus spreading the load.

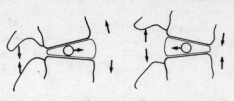

BENDING BACKWARDS   BENDING FORWARD

Figure 6 *The rocking movement when bending:* As we bend forwards and backwards we roll over the nucleus, like a plank over a barrel. A forward bend squeezes the nucleus backwards; bending backwards causes it to move forwards.

The disc is under constant pressure. Professor Alf Nachemson, from Sweden, inserted hollow needles into the third lumbar (low back) disc of questionably willing volunteer students. These needles were connected to a pressure-measuring apparatus. He found that even in the lying position there was considerable internal pressure. The pressure when sitting, particularly if also leaning forwards with no back support, is even higher than when standing. (See Fig. 7.) This must mean that more muscles are working and further compressing the spine when sitting.

Obviously there are reasons for this constant internal disc pressure. A column of blocks of bone separated by elastic mobile joints would tend to be unstable and flop about in all directions. To add stability the blocks of bone are tied to each other by strong semi-elastic ligaments which surround the joints. Because these ligaments are under constant tension they impose a compression force on the disc. To balance this compression force, there must be some way of maintaining pressure within the disc, otherwise it would collapse. To understand the source of this internal pressure it is necessary to know something about the basic nuts and bolts of the chemical structure of the disc.

The disc is about eighty-five per cent water. This is mainly in the centre nucleus and the fluid separating each layer of the annulus. Scattered about in this fluid are specialized living cells called chondrocytes.

All living creatures are made up of collections of cells. In the original single-cell animals this cell had to fulfil all necessary

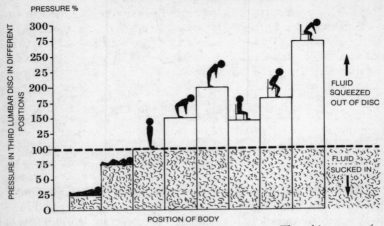

Figure 7 *Pressure inside the disc in various positions:* The white areas of the bar graph above the broken line show body positions (e.g. sitting, bending) in which fluid is squeezed out of the disc. The shaded areas below the line show positions (e.g. lying on one's side) in which fluid is sucked in.

functions to enable life to go on: to digest food, move from A to B, catch food, and so on. It was therefore a very complex single cell.

In time animals became groups of cells, and separate groups of cells within the organism developed special functions, so that some cells took over the sole function of moving the whole from A to B (they became muscles), some took over the function of digestion, and so on. In other words, with increasing complexity of the whole organism, individual cells within each group became more highly specialized so that they could perform only one function amongst many necessary for continued existence. Modern society parallels such changes: with increased complexity the individual contribution to the whole has of necessity become more specialized, so that the functioning of the whole depends on the contribution of an increased number of specialists.

The chondrocytes are one such group of highly specialized cells. Their function is to manufacture one particular chemical compound called a proteoglycan, which they squirt out of their tails. This proteoglycan is structured something like the leaf of a fern (see Fig. 8): the side arms of the 'leaf' are made of a complex sugar compound while the veins of the 'leaf' consist of a protein compound. What is special about this proteoglycan is that each little side branch, because of its chemical structure, carries a negative electrical charge. Similar electrical charges repel each other while opposite charges are attracted to each other. In other words, the similar negatively charged arms are continually trying to push each other away. The force of this repulsion is such that fluid can be held between them whilst under pressure, and this is the source of the internal pressure within the disc. Some plants have utilized a similar internal pressure mechanism and are thus capable of forcing their way even through concrete.

Chondrocytes are living cells and all living cells have to be nourished; they need oxygen and food, and they need to get rid of the wastes produced from the burning up of energy and from their own particular manufacturing process. This is the main function of the circulation, to bring nourishment to the tissues and dispose of wastes. The discs do not have a blood supply

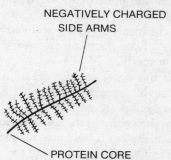

NEGATIVELY CHARGED
SIDE ARMS

PROTEIN CORE

Figure 8 *Proteoglycan:* Specialized cells within the disc (chondrocytes) manufacture the proteoglycan, which is made up of a core of protein with side arms of a sugar. These side arms are negatively charged, and similar electrical charges repel each other. All the closely packed side arms are therefore trying to get away from each other and fluid is trapped between them. This fluid is held there even when the pressure inside the disc is quite high. Proteoglycans are packed tightly together, forming a thick mat. Fluid can only slowly seep through this mat.

within them. The internal pressure is too high for the circulation
to function properly.

Nature, in her usual impeccable manner, has overcome this
problem in an ingenious way. The electrically charged arms of
the proteoglycans are capable of holding fluid under pressure,
depending on the strength of the charge and on how close the
two similar charges are to each other. So if the pressure inside
the disc is below a certain pressure, fluid tends to be sucked into
the disc. Above this level it is squeezed out. The level of pressure
within the disc where fluid is neither sucked in or squeezed out
is that which occurs in the standing position. Referring back to
Professor Nachemson's disc pressure charts (Fig. 7) it is now
possible to see that if we sit down fluid will tend to be squeezed
out of the disc but if we lie down it will tend to be sucked in.
In other words, after a night's sleep we wake up about a centi-
metre taller than when we went to bed, and on the way home
after a day sitting in the office we have to readjust the rear-view
mirror in the car because we have shrunk.

The outer walls of the disc and the cartilage end plate, separating the disc from the bone of the vertebra, act as a sort of
sieve, technically known as a semi-permeable membrane. This
allows water and chemicals up to a certain size to pass through
the sieve, including all the chemicals necessary for the chondrocytes to function properly.

So, nourishment and water can be sucked in and waste products and water can be squeezed out. This is a slow process
because the proteoglycans are packed so closely together. It has
been shown that in the centre of the disc the supply and demand
of chondrocyte nourishment is only just adequate – there is little
to come and go on. This gradual sucking in and squeezing out
of fluid is not in itself sufficient to fulfil the nourishment needs
of the chondrocyte. A further mechanism known as diffusion is
necessary. This is where chemicals in solution tend to spread
from an area of high concentration to areas where the concentration is low. Using oxygen as an example of nourishment and
lactic acid as an example of waste products, it has been shown
(see Fig. 9) that oxygen is in high concentration in the outer

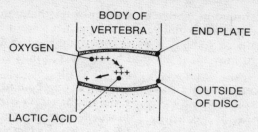

Figure 9 *Diffusion of lactic acid and oxygen within the disc:* The end plates on the top and bottom of each vertebra and the outside of the disc act as a selective sieve. This only allows the necessary ingredients for the nourishment of the chondrocytes to pass through and the waste products of the manufacturing process to pass out. In the centre of the disc the concentration of essential nutrients is only just high enough to maintain the chondrocytes in reasonable health, and the waste disposal system is only just coping. The diagram shows the relative concentrations of oxygen and lactic acid within the discs: more oxygen on the outside than in the centre, and more lactic acid in the centre than on the outside. Without adequate diffusion, assisted by movement, the chondrocytes easily become starved.

parts of the disc and low in the centre, the reverse being so for lactic acid.

The most effective aid to this diffusion is movement, more or less any movement. In other words, our discs were designed for the time when we were more or less always on the move, and we may be starving our chondrocytes by staying in one position too long, whether this be sitting, standing or lying.

The facet joints

The facet joints are designed to limit the movement of the spine to certain directions. The direction of allowed movement depends on how the two joint surfaces are aligned with each other. The movement requirements vary for different regions of the spine, and thus the alignment of these joints also varies.

In the neck maximum mobility is required. Forward looking vision with two eyes has become a necessary part of our survival kit. This limits our field of vision. We need to know what is going on around us, above us and below us, therefore the neck is required to have a full range of movement in all directions. In the low back stability is more important than mobility. The direction of movement allowed by the facet joints is restricted mainly to bending forwards and backwards.

The facet joints also take part in resisting compression and shear stresses, helping to take some of the strain off the discs. (Impact stress is created by a direct pressure at right angles to the surface under stress. Shear stress is created when the pressure is not at right angles to the surface, thus creating a tendency for the applied pressure to shear it off.) This is particularly so in the region of the two reverse curves of the spine: the neck and the low back (see Fig. 10).

These joints are called synovial joints and are constructed like most of the rest of the joints in the body (see Fig. 11). They

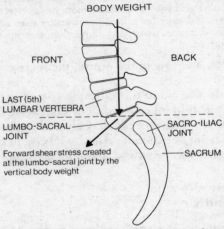

Figure 10 *Compression and shear stress on the joint between the lowest low back vertebra and tail piece:* The pelvis is attached to each side of the tail piece (the sacrum), by means of a strong joint, called the sacro-iliac joint. The joint between the lowest vertebra and the tail piece is called the lumbo-sacral joint. The sacro-iliac joint is behind the lumbo-sacral joint: therefore any downward compression stress will tend to cause a forward shear stress at the lumbo-sacral joint. This will tend to make this joint slip forward. This forward slip is resisted by very strong ligaments and by the angled facet joints.

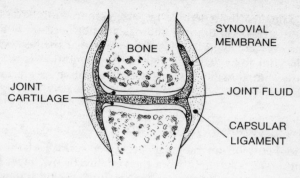

Figure 11 *Cross-section of a typical synovial joint*

have an outer casing, called a capsule. This seals the inside of the joint. Lining the inside of this casing is a layer of specialized cells which manufacture the fluid which lubricates the two surfaces of the joint. Separating the two ends of the joining bones are two thin plates, a few millimetres thick, consisting of tough resilient semi-elastic cartilage, which absorbs any impact, shear, or twisting stresses, thus protecting the ends of the bones. This is possible because it is made up of crisscrossing strands of tough collagen fibres. The cartilage is living tissue and thus gets worn and has to be replaced. Because it is capable of considerable distortion and at times has to carry considerable weight, like the disc it has no blood vessels. Also like the disc this web of collagen fibres contains a scattering of our old friends the chondrocyte cells which manufacture replacement cartilage. These cells are not as far from the surface as in the discs but they still require nourishment, which is provided by the fluid secreted by the specialized cells that line the inside of the capsule, the synovial lining (hence the name for the joints). This fluid therefore has two functions: to transmit nourishment to the chondrocytes and also to lubricate the opposing surfaces of the joint.

If the joint fluid remains stagnant the chondrocytes do not get adequate nourishment, so, also like the discs, frequent movement is necessary for the maintenance of adequate nutrition. Experiments in the laboratory have shown that joint cartilage can be damaged by repetitive impact, compression, stress and also shear stress. Laboratory findings are not necessarily applicable to everyday living but it would seem that the best way to maintain your joint cartilage in a healthy condition is to move frequently, but possibly also to avoid repetitive severe impact and shear stresses.

The neck (cervical) facet joints

When looked at from the side the upper surface of the facet joints in the neck, coming from the vertebra below, faces backwards and upwards. As you go further down the neck they tend to face more backwards and less upwards.

This arrangement has important clinical implications in diagnosing certain neck problems and is also of importance to those who use manipulation. When the neck is bent forward, when we look down, the top surface of the facet joint slides forward on the bottom. Looking from the side it can be seen that this has the effect of enlarging the hole at the side between each vertebra. This is where the nerves exit after leaving the main nerve trunk. If these nerves are being pressed on or irritated by something narrowing this hole, bending the neck forward should therefore give relief. Also, bending the neck backwards, looking up, should have the opposite effect (see Fig. 12).

At the top of the neck where the upper facet joint surface, coming from the vertebra below, faces more upwards than backwards twisting the neck, rotation, will be a more natural movement than side bending. In the lower neck where the joint

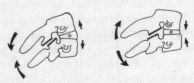

BENDING BACKWARDS   BENDING FORWARD

Figure 12 *Forward and backward bending in the neck:* Note how bending backwards narrows the gap between the facet joints and the disc, where the nerve trunks exit (intervertebral foramen).

surfaces face more backwards than upwards side bending will be easier than twisting (see Fig. 13).

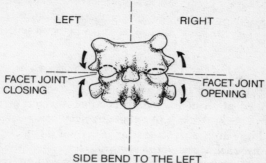

Figure 13 *Back view of the lower neck:* Note how side bending to the left will narrow the exit hole for the nerve roots (intervertebral foramen) on the left and open it up on the right.

When we side bend and rotate the neck to the left the surface of the upper left facet joint will slide down on the lower surface. This will have the effect of closing down on the hole on that side. The opposite will happen on the other side. It is in the lower neck joints where trouble that may involve the nerve roots leaving the spine tends to happen. Therefore painful side bending rather than twisting or rotation of the neck may pinpoint where the trouble lies.

Remember, the neck has a natural reverse curve. Looked at from the side it can be seen (see Fig. 14) that this means the facet joints will have to share some of the load of carrying the head, particularly the upper ones with more horizontal joints.

It can also be seen that the position that would reduce stress on these joints and also keep the side openings less compressed would be the chin tuck-in position with the neck curve as flattened as possible (see Fig. 15). And yet, looking around at one's fellow beings unfortunate enough to be wearing a collar for relief of neck pain, this collar is frequently seen to be high at the front and low at the back. This means that the chin is thrust up, the neck curve is increased, thus further jamming the facet joints into each other. How silly can we get!

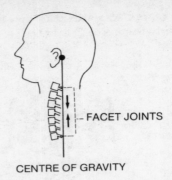

Figure 14 *Side view of the neck showing the centre of gravity:* Note how the facet joints lie in front of the centre of gravity. This means they will have to carry weight.

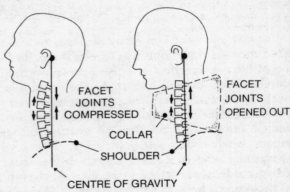

Figure 15 *The correct shape of a neck collar:* A neck collar should be a quarter higher at the back than the front. This unloads the facet joints, brings the neck joints back towards the centre of gravity, and enlarges the intervertebral foramen.

If you have the misfortune to need a collar, see that it is a quarter higher at the back than the front. If it is not, do something about it.

The top two neck vertebrae have their own special characteristics. First, there is no disc between them. The top vertebra, called the atlas, has no body (see Fig. 16). The second vertebra,

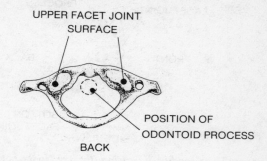

FRONT

UPPER FACET JOINT
SURFACE

POSITION OF
ODONTOID PROCESS

BACK

Figure 16 *The first neck vertebra (the atlas) looked at from above:* There are only two joints attaching it to the skull. These allow free rocking backwards and forwards but no natural twist. This makes it possible to say 'yes' but not 'no'. It has no body. This has been pinched by the second vertebra (the axis).

called the axis, has pinched it. The top vertebra consists of a ring of bone which surrounds the hole in the base of the skull where the main nerve trunk leaves the brain. In some respects it acts like a washer. On its upper surface it has two concave joint surfaces, one on each side. These fit into two knobs on the base of the skull. Because of their shape and position and because there are only two of them, the only natural movement taking place between the skull and the first vertebra is a forward and backward rocking: this is the joint that says 'yes'.

The second vertebra (axis) has a body so that there is a disc between it and the third. Looked at from the side (see Fig. 17) it also has a vertical knob sticking up. This is the body of the first vertebra which it has pinched, and it is called the odontoid process. It locks into the back of the front of the ring of the first vertebra and is tied to it by strong surrounding ligaments. This allows a twisting or rotation movement between it and the first vertebra. At its sides the axis also has the four usual facet joint surfaces, two connecting with the first vertebra and two with the third. The upper joint surfaces are facing nearly vertically upwards and slightly backwards. The natural movement

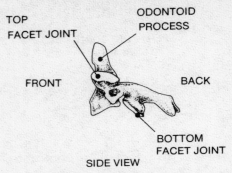

Figure 17 *The second neck vertebra (the axis) looked at from the side:*
The original body of the first vertebra (the odontoid process) sticks up
vertically and forms a joint at the back of the front of the first vertebra.
Combined with the **upward-facing** facet joints this allows free twisting
between the two. The movement between the first and second vertebrae
says 'no', not 'yes'.

allowed by such an arrangement is a rotation, pivoting round
the odontoid process. In other words the joints between the first
and second vertebra play a big part in saying 'no'.

The chest (dorsal or thoracic) facet joints

There are twelve separate blocks of bone, vertebrae, in this part
of the spine. The alignment of the facet joints is a continuation
from those in the lower part of the neck (see Fig. 18). The upper

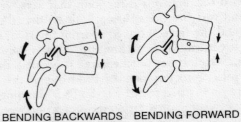

Figure 18 *Side view of the chest (thoracic) spine:* The facet joints are more
backward facing. All movements are restricted because of the attached
rib cage.

surface of the lower joint tends to look more backwards and less upwards, and also slightly sideways, the further down one goes. This allows reasonable freedom in bending forwards, backwards, sideways, and twisting, but to each of these vertebrae is attached a pair of ribs. This restricts all movement and thus stress on the joints. The general shape of this part of the spine, plus the fact that most of it lies behind the centre of gravity, ensures that most of the body weight is carried by the body of the vertebra. Potential stress is thus further reduced on the facet joints.

Painful problems in this part of the spine are less common than in the neck and low back, except at the lowest part. Here there is a sudden change in the alignment of the facet joints. This usually takes place between the twelfth, the last, chest vertebra and the first low back vertebra. The upper joint surface of the first low back vertebra suddenly changes direction from those above, so that it faces inwards and slightly backwards. Such an arrangement on the two sides immediately blocks any twisting or rotation movement.

Lower down the chest the rib cage becomes a less rigid structure. The last two ribs are short and are not joined by bone to the rest of the ribs. This means that more movement is allowed in the lowest two vertebrae, particularly twisting (see Fig. 19).

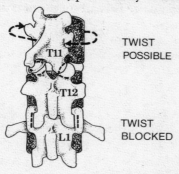

Figure 19 *Back view of the junction between the chest (thoracic) and the low back (lumbar) spine:* Note the sudden change in the alignment of the facet joints of the twelfth (lowest) thoracic vertebra (labelled T12). This allows free twisting in the top joints (between T11 and T12) and none in the bottom joints (between T12 and L1).

But this twisting is suddenly blocked by the change of the alignment of the facet joints between the twelfth chest and first low back vertebrae. Such a sudden change puts a lot of stress on the free-moving parts in any twisting strain. This is the part of the spine that is often overstressed by any movement involving a lot of twisting: a common site of problems in fast bowlers in cricket, professional golfers, baseball batters, and players of any racquet sports. Also, the lower part of the chest spine is vulnerable to another problem very early in life. This will be described later.

The low back (lumbar) facet joints

The alignment of the first low back vertebra facet joints has been described. The upper surface of the facet joint coming from the vertebra below faces inwards. Looked at from above, the front of the surface curves so that it also faces slightly backwards. There is an increasing need for stability rather than mobility in the low back. The bodies of the vertebrae gradually get bigger and the two facet joints at each level get further apart. Gradually the inward-facing facet joint surfaces, coming from the vertebra below, become more backward and slightly upward facing in the lowest part. This arrangement is necessary to resist

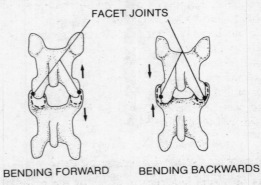

FACET JOINTS

BENDING FORWARD   BENDING BACKWARDS

Figure 20 *Back view of the low back (lumbar) spine:* The alignment of the facet joints allows free bending forward and backwards.

any forward shearing movement of the vertebra above on the one below. This tends to happen because of the reverse curving of the low back spine.

Such an arrangement of the facet joint surfaces allows free forward and backward movement (see Fig. 20). There is some sideways bending possible but rotation or twisting is resisted. That some rotation is possible is because the discs have some give. Also, although we think of bone as hard solid tissue, living bone has in fact a considerable degree of springiness.

The ligaments

The function of ligaments is to add stability to the spine, controlling the range of movement of each joint. They consist of tough collagen fibres that have similar origins to the disc annulus and the joint cartilage, being part of the body's connective or binding tissue. They consist of specialized lengthened cells that have the function of resisting stretch. They have a degree of inbuilt elasticity so that after stretching they return to their original length. Like discs, they are visco-elastic – if only a moderate stretch is maintained for a length of time they do not return immediately to their original length after the stretch is over. It is thus obvious we should not stay in any one position that puts stretch on our ligaments for any length of time: we should keep moving.

When we bend our spine forward, backwards or sideways, the body of the vertebra above rocks over the vertebra below. The pivot point of this rocking motion is approximately the centre of the nucleus of the disc. Ligaments resisting backward bending will therefore be in front of this pivot point, those resisting forward bending will be behind, and those resisting side bend will be on the opposite side to the bend.

Ligaments resisting backward bend

There is only one ligament in front of the pivot of movement. This is a broad strong ligament which surrounds the front of the bodies of the vertebrae and the discs (see Fig. 21). It covers

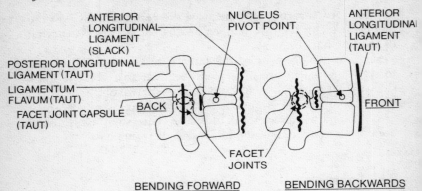

Figure 21 *Side view of the ligaments in the low back (lumbar) spine:*
Bending forwards tightens the ligaments behind the pivot point, the disc nucleus. Bending backwards tightens the ligament in front of the pivot point.

the whole length of the spine and is called the anterior (front) longitudinal ligament. It is firmly attached to the outer wall of the disc and to the middle of the body of the vertebra. This ligament is slack and not at risk when the spine is bent forward, but any backward bending movement, particularly if this is associated with a twist, could lead to possible overstress. This ligament also helps to resist any shearing stress, resisting any tendency for the body of one vertebra to slide forward on the one below.

Ligaments resisting forward bend

There are five ligaments that resist forward bending (see Fig. 22). Working from the pivot point outwards, the one closest to the disc is called the posterior (back) longitudinal ligament. This is attached to the backs of the discs, but not the bodies of the vertebrae, and runs down the whole length of the spine. It is not as broad as the anterior ligament and if the back wall of the disc gives way (ruptures), this tends to happen at the side of the outer limit of this ligament.

The second ligament out from the pivot point is called the

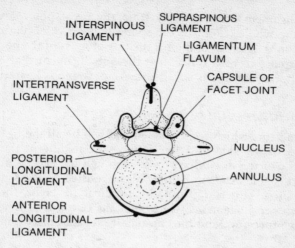

Figure 22 *Cross section of the low back (lumbar) spine showing the ligaments joining each vertebra*

ligamentum flavum (yellow ligament). This lines and joins the front surfaces of the laminae and thus forms a large part of the back wall of the spinal canal, down which the main nerve trunk travels. Not surprisingly, in view of its name, it is more yellow in colour than other ligaments and is also much more elastic. With ageing and shortening of the spine it can thicken and buckle. This may cause some obstruction in the main spinal canal.

The third ligaments out are those surrounding the casing (capsule) of the facet joints. The fibres in this casing are not arranged up and down but tend to criss-cross each other. They are therefore not efficient resisters of straight forward bending. Their ability to resist forward bending depends on their ability to resist extremes of movement within the facet joints themselves.

The fourth ligaments from the pivot point are those that tie the individual spinous processes together, one at each side and one straight behind. They are called the intertransverse and interspinous ligaments. The ones joining the side arms, the intertransverse, will also resist side bend.

The ligament furthest away from the pivot point stretches down the whole length of the spine. It is an extension of the interspinous ligament and joins the tips of most of the posterior (back) spines to each other. It is the only ligament that can be felt from the outside. It is called the supraspinous ligament.

Ligaments resisting side bend

The ligaments which resist a side bend will be all the ligaments that are to the side of a line joining the middle of the front and back of the disc which passes through the centre of pivot. Therefore, side bend to the left will be resisted by the right half of the broad anterior (front) longitudinal ligament, the right intertransverse ligaments which joins the two side arms (lateral spinous processes), and the capsule of the right facet joint.

All this may seem a lot of unnecessary detail but in fact ligaments can get overstrained and to understand how to avoid this it is necessary to know how they work and what they do. Ligaments furthest away from the pivot point will be more vulnerable to strain: the effect of leverage will be greatest. The maximum stress in bending forward will fall on the posterior interspinous and supraspinous ligaments. Post mortem studies have shown that scarring, indicating previous injury, is quite common in these ligaments.

So often, attacks of back pain are caused by a forward bend with a twist in it. When we bend forward the ligaments behind the pivot point tighten up (see Fig. 23). If we then side bend to the left these tight ligaments will tend to be further tightened on the right side. To reduce this increased tension on the right side the spine will naturally want to twist to the right – the opposite way to the side bend. This is not what happens when we bend to pick up something to one side of us: we bend forward, side bend, and also twist towards the object we wish to pick up. This puts tremendous stress on the ligaments on the opposite side, in particular the capsules of the facet joints. Post mortem studies have shown these facet joint capsules to be a common site of previous injuries.

To reduce the risk of injury to these ligaments when bending and lifting it is now obvious that as little of the necessary movement as is possible should be done by the spine. This means that the hips and knees should be bent, not the spine. Also, the object needing lifting should be faced as square on as is possible.

From what has so far been said there are two clear messages. To keep one's spine from getting prematurely old requires plenty of movement. Try not to sit for too long watching things happening – get up and make them happen. Also, if you have to bend, do it with your hips and knees, not your back.

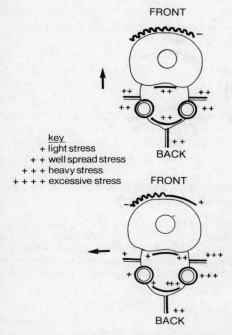

FORWARD BEND

FRONT

BACK

key
+ light stress
+ + well spread stress
+ + + heavy stress
+ + + + excessive stress

FRONT

BACK

FORWARD BEND & LEFT SIDE BEND

Figure 23

FORWARD BEND & LEFT SIDE BEND
& RIGHT ROTATION

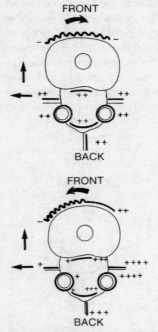

FORWARD BEND & LEFT SIDE BEND
& LEFT ROTATION

Figure 23 (cont.) *The effect of forward and side bending and twisting on the ligaments of the low back:* Forward bending, side bending one way, and twisting the other, naturally spreads the strain on the low back ligaments. Forward bending and then side bending and twisting the same way puts the ligaments at risk on the opposite side to the bend and twist.

The muscles

Our muscles provide the means whereby we can act on the information we have received from our sensory or sensing system. They give us the ability to act on the information received, the power of movement that is allowed by our system of joints.

The basic unit of the muscle is a highly specialized cell called a muscle fibre. Its only function is to shorten, contract, or lengthen. Each muscle fibre consists of a complex organic structure arranged like the interlocking of the tines of two forks (see Fig. 24). Each tine is connected to the tine of the other fork by fine filaments. Each fibre is connected to the nerve ending of a so-called motor nerve, which is essential to its existence. In fact the muscle fibre could be considered as a highly specialized ending to the nerve: when the nerve is cut and dies the muscle fibre dies.

When the motor nerve fires off a message it initiates a chemical reaction within the muscle fibre that has the effect of shortening the connecting links between the tines of the two forks. This draws one fork towards the other: in other words, shortens the muscle fibre.

The motor nerve, like other nerves, is a highly specialized cell

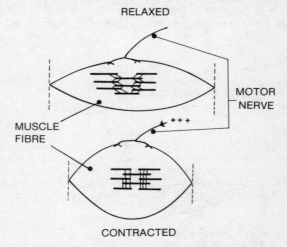

RELAXED

MOTOR
NERVE

MUSCLE
FIBRE

CONTRACTED

Figure 24 *A muscle fibre contracting:* Firing of the motor nerve initiates a chemical reaction within the muscle fibre which has the effect of shortening the links between each muscle filament, thus shortening the whole muscle fibre.

which has the ability to transmit a message along its fibre by means of an electro-chemical reaction. This can be detected as an electric current running along the fibre. The motor nerve cell body lies in the spinal cord, in the spinal canal, and the long fibre coming from the body travels down in a nerve going to the muscle (see Fig. 25). Each motor nerve fibre divides into several branches within the muscle. The ending of each branch supplies one individual muscle fibre.

Muscle fibres vary in size within a limited range. The thickness of each motor nerve fibre also varies within a limited range. As a general rule the thinnest nerve fibres split up into the smallest number of branches and supply the smallest-sized muscle fibres. Conversely, the thickest nerve fibres split up into the greatest number of branches and supply the largest-sized muscle fibres.

The smaller-sized muscle fibres are called red muscle fibres and the larger are called white fibres. The smaller red muscle fibres have a richer blood supply.

As a general rule when effort is required the smaller-sized muscle fibres are stimulated first. When more effort is needed the larger sizes are brought into action. The smaller red muscle

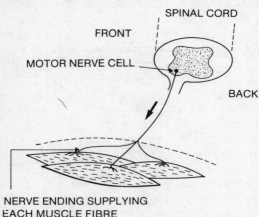

Figure 25 *A motor nerve supplying the muscle fibres:* Each motor nerve branches inside the muscle and connects with several muscle fibres. The larger the nerve cell and nerve fibre the more individual muscle fibres supplied.

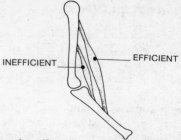

Figure 26 *Efficient and inefficient muscle action:* The closer the origin and insertion of a muscle is to the joint it moves the less efficient it becomes in moving that joint.

fibres are capable of more prolonged action, while the larger white fibres, though stronger, get fatigued more easily.

Different muscles have to fulfil different functional needs: some are needed for occasional strong action, others are needed for continuous action to help counter gravity, keeping us on our feet or seat.

Those needing to be in action most of the time are called postural muscles. Those required for intermittent stronger action, to get us from A to B, are called phasic muscles. As a general rule the postural muscles contain a higher percentage of red fibres. Because each individual motor nerve supplying the red fibres has fewer branches, finer tuning of activity is possible.

To move a joint the muscle needs to be attached to the bones on each side of the joint. These attachments are known as the origin and the insertion. For the sake of convenience the attachment nearest to the head is called the origin and the attachment furthest from the head the insertion.

These attachments are usually by means of a strong semi-elastic tendon which is a continuation of the casing of the muscle fibres.

Some muscles cross just one joint so that when these muscles contract only that one joint is moved. Others cross several joints so that contraction of the muscle effects movement of them all.

The further away the origin and insertion of the muscle from the joint to be moved, the more effective is the muscle in moving that joint (see Fig. 26).

Muscles of the neck and back

The muscles of the neck and back are arranged in three layers on each side of the spine. The pivot point of movement in the spine is the disc nucleus. All muscles behind that point will therefore pull the spine backwards when they contract on both sides.

The deepest layer consists of small insignificant muscles which join one vertebra to the next. When those on each side contract together they pull just one vertebra backwards on the next one – thus locally extending just two units of the whole spine.

The middle layer of muscles usually spans between two and four vertebrae, so that when they contract together on both sides of the spine all of the joints they span will be pulled backwards.

The outer layer of muscles, the ones which can be felt from the outside, span several vertebrae. The ones in the neck travel from the base of the skull as far as the upper part of the chest area of the spine, while those covering the low back stretch from the upper part of the chest spine as far as the tail piece. They are long and relatively narrow muscles.

The main back muscles therefore have the following characteristics: they are postural muscles, more or less constantly active; they are close to the joints they move, and are therefore not very efficient movers of those joints; they are long and thin and therefore not designed as strength muscles, but they do have a relatively large range of movement.

Postural muscles, due to their constant activity, have a tendency to shorten and tighten if they are not stretched out regularly, while phasic muscles if not used regularly tend to get weak and flabby.

It should now be evident that our back muscles need regular stretching, and that shortening, strengthening exercises are not helpful.

It should also be evident that when we do any lifting, particularly with our arms well away from our bodies, the effort needed to pull our spines backwards would be an excessive strain on these back muscles and that they will need any help they can get. A lot of this help comes from the abdominal muscles. These will be described in detail later.

The nerves

To understand neck and back problems it is necessary to have a working knowledge of how parts of our nervous system work. It is not necessary to understand the finer details of how nerves transmit messages but it is necessary to appreciate that when a nerve cell is stimulated to fire off, a chemically induced electric current travels along the nerve fibre. This is the same for all nerves whatever part they play in the overall scheme of things.

Each nerve cell is highly specialized to fulfil one function only, to transmit this electro-chemical message along the length of its fibre.

Basically, the nervous system consists of an ingoing sensory or sensing system and an outgoing action or motor system. At the centre of the nervous sytem is the brain, which is a sort of computer made up of millions upon millions of nerve cells receiving, translating and transmitting messages. The brain is connected to the rest of the body by the spinal cord. This travels down the canal in the spine which lies behind the body of each vertebra.

If a cut is taken straight across this spinal cord it will be seen to consist of a central part called the grey matter and an outer part called the white matter. The grey matter consists of masses of nerve cells while the white matter consists of columns of nerve fibres.

The spinal cord ends at about the level of the second of the five low back vertebrae and the canal below this level is filled with nerve roots travelling down to the lower parts of the body.

We have evolved from a segmental design. This means that nerves exit and enter at each separate segment, passing through the openings (foramen) at the side between adjacent vertebrae, each nerve supplying a specific segment of the body.

At each segmental level of the spinal cord four nerve roots emerge, two from each side. The ones at the front are called the anterior and the ones at the back the posterior (see Fig. 27). The front roots contain the motor nerve fibres, going to the body's muscles. The ones at the back contain the sensory nerve fibres. There is a bulge (ganglion) on these posterior roots. This bulge houses the sensory nerve cell bodies. The motor nerve cell bodies lie in the front part of the grey matter of the spinal cord. These two nerve roots unite before they pass out through bony canals at the sides of the spine. The united nerve root thus contains both sensory and motor nerve fibres.

Shortly after leaving the spine this main nerve root divides into a front (anterior) and a back (posterior) branch. It is this posterior branch that supplies the main back muscles and joints.

With the evolutionary development of the arms and legs this

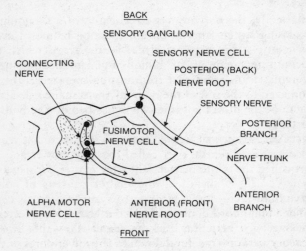

Figure 27 *Cross section of the main nerve trunk (spinal cord):* This shows the reflex connections between the incoming messages in the sensing (sensory) nerves and the outgoing messages through the two types of motor nerves (the fusimotor and alpha).

segmental arrangement has become a bit complicated. The muscles moving the arms and legs cross more than one segment and therefore each nerve supplying the muscles contains nerve fibres coming from more than one root. In the regions of the spine from which the nerve supply to the arms and legs arises, there is an intermingling of the nerve roots shortly after they leave the spine. This region of intermingling is called the cervical plexus in the neck, and the lumbar plexus in the low back.

This mixing up of the nerve roots ensures that each separate nerve leaving the plexus contains fibres that have come from more than one segmental nerve root.

This complicated arrangement ensures that people such as neurologists earn their keep. If a nerve root is damaged at or near the spine so that motor nerves are damaged this will lead to loss of strength in those muscles that derive some of their nerve supply from that particular segmental level. If you have a muscle supplied by branches from three or four levels it can be very difficult to sort out which level is responsible for the weakness.

There is another complication in the neck region. During evolution, to ensure freedom of neck movement, the arm buds have moved down the spine, so that the arms are attached more to the upper part of the chest. The nerves supplying the arms were also dragged down, so that muscles moving the shoulders and arms derive their nerve supply from the neck segments. But some of the muscles that move the shoulder girdle are attached to the chest wall. This means a pain in the chest region may in fact come from trouble in the neck.

Sensory nerves

We are aware of many different sensations, such as touch, heat, cold and pain. All nerves transmit the same electro-chemical message. To help the brain interpret the signals received the sensory nerves have developed specialized endings in the tissues supplied by them, so that only one particular stimulus can fire off one particular nerve ending. This encoding allows the brain to make the correct interpretation of the incoming message.

The thickness of the sensory nerve fibres varies within a small range. The speed of travel of any message along the nerve fibre varies with the thickness of the fibre: the thicker the nerve fibre the more rapid is transmission of the electro-chemical message.

There is an inbuilt pecking order within this sensing system, so that messages coming through the large-fibred sensing nerves tend to block out, inhibit, the messages coming through the smaller. As a general rule the larger-fibred nerves have endings that are stimulated by the more pleasant sensations, such as touch and gentle pressure, while endings associated with more unpleasant sensations have the smaller fibres. Those associated with the sensation of pain have the smallest fibres.

This means that if we stimulate the larger-fibred nerves we can block off the input from the smaller. In other words, pain can be kissed or stroked away. All parents know this.

To enable incoming messages to reach the brain it is necessary to have a series of links between nerve fibres. Sensations have a long way to travel from different parts of the body, so that messages have to be passed along a chain of nerve cells and their fibres. The incoming message is passed between each nerve by special chemicals called neuro-transmitters. The incoming signal causes a slight chemical change in the transmitter which is then able to fire off the next nerve cell. It is at these junctions between nerves that incoming messages can be modified, either enhanced or inhibited, by messages coming from other nerve cells and also by chemicals and drugs in the surrounding tissue fluid that have got there by means of the blood stream.

The sensory nerve endings have a varying ability to adapt. This means if the nerve endings are stimulated by the appropriate sensation for a length of time the nerve eventually stops firing. For instance, if you are touched in a particular area you are immediately aware of that touch. If the touching remains in the same place it is not long before you are no longer aware of that touch. This fact is worth knowing in any form of body contact: keep those hands moving.

Some nerve endings adapt more quickly than others. The nerves ultimately responsible for the sensation of pain do not adapt at all: once they are fired off they keep on firing until the stimulation is removed. This is to be expected: we need to know if something is continuing to hurt us to encourage action to remove the hurt.

The skin and surface tissue sensing nerves have to do with contact with the outside world. Deeper tissues also have their own specialized sensing nerves. Our main concern is with those in the muscles and joint casings.

All sensory nerves have a connection to the motor nerve cell which lies in the spinal cord. Incoming sensations can either excite or inhibit (relax) the motor nerve. Those that excite the motor nerve make it more likely to fire off and those that inhibit make it less likely. The more pleasant sensations will tend to make us want to stick around and enjoy them, while unpleasant ones will tend to stimulate the desire to remove ourselves. In other words, the input from larger-fibred sensing nerves inhibits the motor nerve while the input from the smaller tends to excite.

Pain nerves

The appreciation of pain is a subjective emotion which may be influenced by many factors in our lives. The sensing nerves in our tissues capable of causing this feeling of pain are widely distributed throughout the body: skin, muscles, joints, and so on.

These pain nerves, called nociceptors (noxious receptors), have the smallest diameter nerve fibres and end in simple fine filaments. They are fired off by unpleasant (noxious) sensations, as happens when our tissues are injured. This stimulation may be chemical or mechanical. The chemical stimulation comes from substances that are released when tissue is damaged and when the healing process is taking place. It can also come from tissue that is not getting rid of its wastes adequately, as may happen in muscle that is in spasm and is fatigued.

The mechanical stimulation comes from distortion of the nerve endings as could happen if the endings were stretched by injury to the tissue containing them.

It is important to bear in mind that, whatever the stimulus, these pain nerves keep on firing until that stimulus is removed. They fire until the reaction to injury, the healing process, has returned the tissue to normal; or until a muscle in painful spasm becomes relaxed; or until anything distorting the nerve ending stops distorting it.

It is necessary to know which tissues in the back are supplied by pain nerve endings and which are not.

Pain nerve endings are found in most of the tissues surrounding the back and neck joints: in the muscles, the muscle tendons, the ligaments, joint casings, the surface of the discs, the linings of the bones, and the linings of the blood vessels that supply the joints, bones and muscles.

They are not found in the lining of the inside of the joints (synovial lining), or in the cartilage separating the two bony surfaces of the facet joints, or in the back of the lining surrounding the spinal canal (called the dura). This is why it is possible to use a needle to tap the fluid surrounding the spinal cord from behind without too much discomfort.

The nerve endings are also not found in the middle of the disc. They have been found penetrating the outer layers of the annulus but it is not sure how functional such endings are: they are in tissue that is under constant internal pressure. It is possible that they are just non-functioning remnants from an earlier stage of development.

This is important information: ageing, wear and tear, of the disc starts in the middle – thus quite a lot of this wear and tear can happen before there are any painful consequences.

The wide distribution of pain nerve endings explains why it is virtually impossible to define where the pain is coming from when our necks or backs hurt. As mentioned before, if we move a joint and it hurts we can say with reasonable certainty this is where the pain is coming from. It is very difficult to move one vertebra on another without moving others in the vicinity, and it is impossible to move one of the three joints between each vertebra without moving the other two. Things are made more difficult because we are dealing with joints well under the surface of the skin in the low back.

The type of pain experienced is also of little help in defining the source. Wherever the pain nerves are fired off the signal travelling up the nerve fibre is the same. That some pain is experienced as knife-like, burning, aching, or whatever, depends on the brain's interpretation of this pain, not on where it is coming from.

The thickness (diameter), of the pain nerves varies within a small range. The thicker-fibred nerves are called 'fast' pain nerves, and the thinner are called 'slow' pain nerves (see Fig. 28). The fast pain nerves are designed for emergencies: the nerve fibres are longer, they have less junctions to cross on their way to the brain, and because of the thicker fibre the message travels faster. The resulting pain is experienced as sudden and sharp and it stimulates reflex withdrawal of the painful part: we get

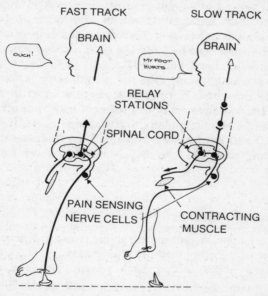

Figure 28 *Fast and slow pain nerves:* The fast pain nerves are larger than the slow. The larger the diameter of a nerve fibre the more rapid is the transmission of messages. The fast pain nerves have less relay stations on the way to the brain. But the first line of defence is the reflex connections which all pain nerves have with motor nerves to associated muscles. Reflex connections go *directly* to the muscle (they do not involve the brain), so that rapid action can be taken to get away from the source of the pain.

out of the way without having to think about it. The input from the 'slow' pain nerves has several junctions to cross. As already mentioned, it is at these junctions where the incoming messages may be modified: either enhanced or suppressed.

Nature has placed a further obstacle to our ability to define the source of our neck and back pain. The pain nerves supplying the joints and surrounds of each separate vertebra in the neck and lower back do not arise only from that particular segment. They travel up and down so that nerves coming from one segment supply at least three adjacent segments. This means that when our brain interprets pain as coming from one particular site this may in fact not be its real source.

The pain caused by stimulation of the nerves in our spines has a deep, ill-defined quality: we try and locate it with our hands rather than our fingers. This ill-defined pain may spread out from the spine and be experienced in various parts of our head, shoulders, arms, rump, thighs, and legs. This is what is known as a *referred* pain – the brain misinterprets its source. This has to do with our original segmental structure so that pain stimulated in any part of one segment may appear to come from any other part stimulated by the same segment. This is further confused in the neck and low back because the pain nerves at any particular site may come from several different segments.

Muscle sensing nerves

Our muscles contain two different highly specialized sensing nerves. One of these is called the muscle spindle. These spindles are scattered about within each muscle and the number contained in each muscle varies. This seems to depend on the function of each particular muscle.

The other specialized sensing nerve lies in the tendons at each end of the muscle and is called a Golgi tendon organ (named after the scientist who first described it).

Muscle spindle The spindles are scattered about within the

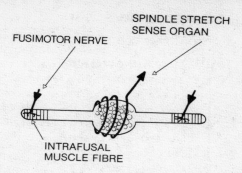

Figure 29 *A very much simplified muscle spindle:* The fusimotor nerve supplies the muscle fibres at each end of the spindle.

muscle so that they act in series. Their sole function is to monitor any lengthening or shortening of the whole muscle.

It is a highly complex structure (see Fig. 29) but in essence consists of a sensing nerve ending which is coiled round the centre part of a tube. When this centre part is stretched out, as will happen when the muscle lengthens, the coils of the sensing nerve are stretched apart. This stimulates them to fire off. Each end of the spindle consists of fine muscle fibres. These muscle fibres are fired off by a separate motor nerve to that which fires off the main muscle. The motor nerves firing off the spindle muscles are much smaller than the ones supplying the main muscles and are part of a system called the fusimotor nerves. If these fusimotor nerves fire off it will have the effect of pulling apart the centre of the spindle, stretching the sensing nerve endings which will thus fire them off (see Fig. 30). In other words, the sensing nerves can be fired off not only by lengthening of the whole muscle but also by activity in the muscles at each end of the spindle (see Fig. 31).

This means that there is a fine tuning mechanism within the muscle so that messages can be passed back from the muscle, whatever length it is functioning at.

When the main (Alpha) motor nerve is instructed to fire off (thus shortening the muscle) the fusimotor nerves are also instructed to fire off. This is called a co-activation. It means that

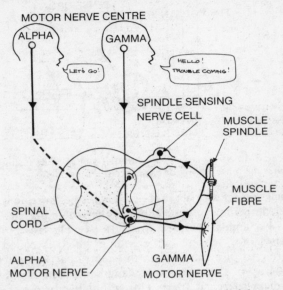

Figure 30 *The connections of the fusimotor (gamma) and alpha motor nerves:* The fusimotor (gamma) nerves are part of our alerting system. When danger threatens they are fired off. This contracts the ends of the spindles. This fires off the stretch-sensing nerve on the middle of the spindle. This relays a message back to the main muscle motor nerve. This primes the muscle motor nerve so that when action is decided such action is facilitated.

as the whole muscle shortens the centre of the spindle is kept at a constant length by the associated shortening of the muscles at each end of the spindle.

As with all sensing nerves the muscle spindle nerve cell lies in the ganglion, swelling, in the posterior nerve root just before it joins the spinal cord. It sends off a nerve fibre back into the spinal cord and from there makes connections with other nerve cells which relay the message back to the central computer — the brain. The incoming message is also relayed directly to the muscle motor nerve which is connected to the muscle concerned, and the message has an exciting effect. This means that if there

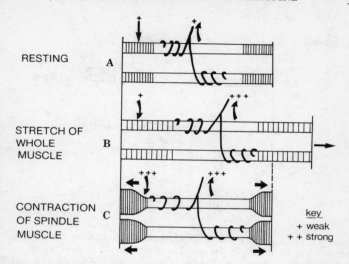

RESTING   A

STRETCH OF
WHOLE   B
MUSCLE

CONTRACTION   C
OF SPINDLE
MUSCLE

key
+ weak
+ + strong

Figure 31 *Stimulation of the stretch-sensitive nerves of the muscle spindle:* The stretch-sensing nerves of the muscle spindles may be fired off either by stretch of the whole muscle or by contraction of the muscle at each end of the spindle.

is a sudden lengthening of a muscle the motor nerve is excited – thus stimulating the muscle to shorten back to its original length.

It is this circuit that is being tested when, for instance, the knee is tapped by a doctor's rubber hammer (see Fig. 32). When the tendon below the kneecap is tapped it imparts a sudden stretch to the muscle in front of the thigh. This stretches the spindles in that muscle and the spindle sensing nerves are fired off. This excites the motor nerve to that muscle which then fires off. This makes the muscle suddenly contract causing the knee to straighten suddenly.

If there is a break anywhere in this circuit the tap on the tendon will fail to fire off the muscle. This break occasionally happens where the motor nerve fibres pass out from the spinal cord just before tey leave the spine through the openings at the sides. It is here that a lump of disc material that has ruptured can damage the root containing the motor nerve fibres.

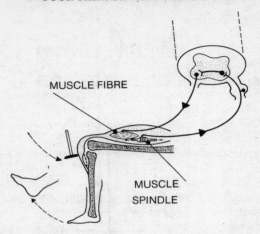

MUSCLE FIBRE

MUSCLE
SPINDLE

Figure 32 *The knee jerk reflex:* Tapping the tendon below the kneecap causes a minute stretch to the spindles in the muscle in front of the thigh. This fires off the stretch-sensing spindle nerve. This relays a message back to the muscle motor nerve. This fires off, making the muscle contract, thus jerking the leg forward.

Golgi tendon organs These sensing nerves have highly specialized endings which lie in the tendons at each end of the muscles. Unlike the spindles they lie parallel to each other. Their sole function is to measure tension in the tendon and thus in the muscle. If this tension reaches high levels, when the muscle is being asked to do more than is reasonable, these endings are fired off. They also have a direct link with the motor nerve that drives that particular muscle, but their effect on the motor nerve is opposite to that of the spindle nerve: they dampen or inhibit its action, thus slackening off the muscle and reducing the tension.

Joint sensing nerves

The casing of most of our synovial joints contain a highly complex system of sensing nerve endings. To understand what may have gone wrong when our necks or backs hurt it is necessary to know something about them.

The casing of our spinal facet joints contains up to four different sensing nerve endings. These are graded according to the thickness of their nerve fibres and they fulfil different functions which are determined by the specialized structure of their endings (see Fig. 33).

The thinnest-fibred nerves are the pain nerves which have been described.

The next in size, called Type 1, have specialized endings which are sensitive to tension within the casing of the joint: tension that is constantly present and also tension created by movement of the joint. These nerves have a low threshold for activity, which means they are easily fired off. Recordings from nerves supplying joints have shown that some of them are firing off even when the joint is at rest.

In the spinal cord the fibres of these particular nerves have a

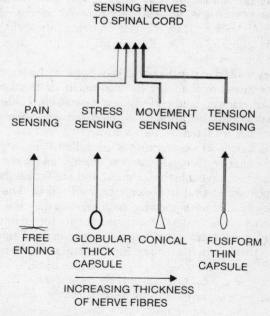

Figure 33 *The joint sensing nerves*

hot line, reflex connections, to the fusimotor nerves rather than to the main (called Alpha) motor nerves.

This means that when they are firing off the fusimotor nerve is excited. This in turn causes increased activity in the muscles at the ends of the spindle. This, in turn, tends to excite the main motor nerve making it more likely to fire off.

Those of us unfortunate enough to have worn arthritic joints can often tell when the weather is changing and it is going to rain by the increased stiffness and soreness in our joints.

There is a simple reason for this. Inside our sealed joints there is a constant negative atmospheric pressure. A change in the outside atmospheric pressure will therefore alter the tension in the capsule of the joint which separates the two different pressures. This will fire off more of these Type 1 nerve endings, which in turn will fire off more of the fusimotor nerves. This in turn will make the muscle spindles more sensitive to stretch, giving the sense of stiffness. It will also provoke increased painful contraction within the muscles moving the joint. These invariably contain potentially painful so-called trigger points. More about these later.

The next sized nerve fibres called Type 2, have specialized endings which are fired off by movement of the joint. They signal the beginning and end of joint movement. Little seems to be known about their central connections and their effect on the motor nerves seems to be variable.

The thickest joint sensing nerves are called Type 3. They have endings similar to the Golgi tendon organs, and have the same function. They have a high threshold and are thus only fired off when the joint casing is under increased stress. They tell the muscles the joints have gone far enough, thus they inhibit rather than excite muscle activity. Type 3 nerves are found in the casing of the low back facet joints but not in the neck. This probably relates to the fact that mobility is more important than stability in the neck, the reverse applying in the low back.

The motor nerves

There are three separate motor systems that respond to incoming sensations.

The first is called the autonomic (automatic) nervous system. This system regulates body functions well beyond conscious control, such as digestion, heart rate, and so on.

It is divided into what are called sympathetic and parasympathetic nerves. These two types of nerves tend to have opposite effects. As far as the neck and back are concerned it is the effects of the sympathetic nerves that is of most interest. This system is automatically fired off when there is an input from a noxious stimulation firing off the pain nerves. They cause us to break out in a cold sweat. In other words they stimulate the sweat glands. More important, they stimulate fine muscles in the walls of blood vessels, making them contract. This has the effect of cutting down the blood supply to the skin and muscles. When pain has been going on for some time this effect can be quite local. It can be detected by using a machine capable of measuring the skin's resistance to an electric current. If an area of skin is found to have an increased resistance to the current it shows that there is increased sympathetic activity in that area.

By using such a machine it is often possible, in those who have suffered neck or back pain of some duration, to detect many small areas of skin with an increased resistance to an electric current. These areas relate to underlying so-called muscle trigger points and also to the sites of traditional Chinese acupuncture points. More will be said of this later.

The main (Alpha) motor nerves We have already (page 46) seen how the final pathway to the muscle comes from the nerve cell which resides in the front part of the grey matter of the spinal cord (see Fig. 27). Each motor nerve cell has multiple connections coming to it from the terminal fibres of sensing nerves. These connections can either excite the motor nerve, making it more likely to fire off, or inhibit it, making it less likely to fire off. The ultimate command to fire off comes from a nerve fibre connection arising from a nerve cell residing in the brain, from an area known as the motor cortex.

In the process of learning how to control our muscles so that they fire off in the right sequence to achieve the desired movement we have to learn to inhibit the firing of muscles not necessary for that movement. The change from the haphazard movements of the newborn to the controlled movement of the adult is due to our ability to learn how to fire off the right muscles at the right time and to cut out any unnecessary firing in the rest of the muscles. The more skilled we become in any particular activity the less muscle effort is required. All unnecessary muscle activity is inhibited in the process of learning so that any highly skilled movement has the maximum economy of movement. Such fine control reaches its peak in, for example, concert pianists.

This means that any influence, for example from the sensing nerves coming in to the motor nerve, can be suppressed, so that the motor nerve will only fire off when so commanded by the central programmed computer in the brain.

An example of this control is shown by a technique known as bio-feedback. By means of fine wire electrodes it is possible to tap a single motor nerve to a muscle and record its firing activity. This activity is converted into a visual or sound signal. It is possible for most individuals to learn how to fire off this single motor nerve at will and to suppress activity in all the rest. Such a technique can be used to teach people how to relax their muscles effectively. This works very well with muscles that are already used to skilled movements, such as those in the forearm. It is a different story when dealing with the more central muscles, particularly those in our necks and backs. This poorly developed inhibitory control is the reason why these muscles tend to get uptight when we get uptight.

The fusimotor nerves   These are the motor nerves which drive the small muscles at each end of the spindles. Their nerve cells reside in the grey matter of the spinal cord, behind those of the main alpha motor nerve cells (see Fig. 27). They are smaller than the alpha motor nerves and the central control area is in a lower, more primitive region of the brain.

Most research into the fusimotor system has been performed on animals which had had their main nerve trunks severed (decerebrate). Until recently it was impossible to record and measure activity in this sytem in conscious human beings. In animals it has been found that this motor system is constantly active, even when the rest of the muscle is relaxed. In animals it provides an essential feedback of information from the muscle spindles, enabling efficient control of muscle activity, at varying degrees of stretch.

Recent research in humans has shown little or no activity in the fusimotor nerves within the muscles of the forearm when the subject consciously relaxes. This suggests the fusimotor system has become less important in the general scheme of things, and that improved central control of movement has made it superfluous in humans. We have learned to think before we act, sometimes.

Information passed back from the spindle to the spinal cord, exciting the main motor nerve to a greater or lesser extent, is capable of little if any influence on the motor nerve in any programmed learned movement. The pattern of firing is present in the central computer of the brain.

The feedback through the fusimotor system may still play a part in the initial process of learning a skilled movement: a tuned constant feedback may tell the central computer if a planned movement is or is not going according to requirement.

It would thus seem the fusimotor system has to some extent become defunct: a sort of appendix in the nervous system.

The fusimotor system is also an active part of our primitive alerting system: if we are threatened, uptight, anxious, there is increased activity in the fusimotor nerves supplying all our muscles. This has the effect of priming up our muscle spindles and thus heightening the sensitivity of our main motor nerves, getting us ready for a quick exit. In the muscles of our arms, for example, this will have little outward effect, except to make them a bit more sensitive to the command to fire off, but in the more central muscles, particularly those in the neck and back

where there is less well developed central control, the effect can
be dramatic. The muscles become tense and tight. In other
words, if we become uptight our neck and back muscles also
become uptight. This can easily lead to a pain – muscle spasm
– pain cycle, which in itself can become self perpetuating. It is
no coincidence that our necks and backs tend to 'go out' at the
times when we are under increased stress.

Another part of our alerting system is a general sense of
wakefulness: we become keyed up and alert, ready to cope with
imminent dangers. This effect shows up in our sleep pattern:
our sleep becomes shallow; we are more easily wakened and
have difficulty getting back to sleep; we wake earlier in the
morning. Really deep restorative sleep is known as Phase 4
sleep. The time spent in this Phase 4 sleep is lessened. We
therefore tend to wake up tired and listless.

If this is happening it is time to take notice and try to do
something about the stresses provoking too much activity in our
alerting system, to avoid the risk of our neck or back giving
trouble.

Pain

The important aspects of the nervous system relating to our
necks and backs have been described. It is now possible to go
back and fill in more details about pain, its side effects, and
how it can be modified.

If someone tells me they have a pain I believe them. It is very
rare for a pain to be completely imaginary. Some pain nerve
endings are being fired off somewhere by something, and
because of their inability to adapt, they will keep on firing until
the source of their irritation goes away by itself or is removed.
If someone tells you no cause can be found for your pain and
that you must be imagining it, invariably the fault lies with the
examiner's inability to detect the source, not in your imagination. Somewhere there is inflammation, a reaction to injury,
local muscle in spasm, or distorted pain nerve endings.

There are three types of pain experienced by those suffering from neck and back problems: local pain, referred pain, and nerve root pain. Local and referred pain have already been described (page 52). The local pain has a deep ill-defined quality and is located by using the hand rather than a finger. The referred pain also has an ill-defined quality and often there is a patchy spread down the arms or legs.

Local and referred pain may also be associated with sensations of numbness, coldness, or pins and needles. These sensations are often felt further down the limb than the pain. For instance, the pain may be felt down the thigh but the pins and needles are experienced in the foot and toes. These sensations are not due to a trapped nerve but to one of the reflex effects of stimulation of pain nerve endings. Messages passing along their fibres are seemingly capable of modifying the input from other sensing nerves. If a sensing nerve fibre is trapped and damaged the input through the nerve is blocked. This results in complete loss of sensation, anaesthesia, not a feeling of altered sensation.

Nerve root pain is provoked when the nerve root is involved in some reaction to injury, usually just before it exits from the sides of the spine. In the low back this is usually due to a rupturing of the disc. The piece of ruptured disc may press on and irritate the nerve root, provoking a reaction to injury. This results in a more severe and unremitting local pain and a severe continuous pain spreading down the arm or leg.

The discs in the low back most likely to give way are those subject to most stress – the lower two. Usually, but by no means always, the pain spreading from the lowest disc when it ruptures goes into the back of the rump, the back of the thigh and calf, the heel, the outside of the foot, and sometimes as far as the little toe. When the next disc up has given way the pain goes from the rump to the outside of the back of the thigh, the outside of the calf, across to the top and inside of the foot, and sometimes as far as the big toe. Later, we will discuss in greater detail how to diagnose your own ruptured disc.

The discs in the neck rarely rupture but the lower ones are sometimes subject to rapid wear and tear which can lead to nerve root pain. This is a severe pain spreading in a continuous

line down the arm as far as the thumb and or some of the
fingers.

When the nerve roots are irritated there will also be widespread irritation of other pain nerves round the back of the disc,
so in the presence of nerve root pain there will also be local and
probably referred pain.

When pain nerves are fired off this signifies tissue injury. This
triggers off reflex effects, effects beyond conscious control, in
order to minimize that injury and to protect the injured part.

As it enters the spinal cord each incoming pain nerve fibre
makes a connection, either directly or indirectly, with each of
the three effector motor nerve systems.

The autonomic sympathetic nerves are excited. This has the
effect of contracting the blood vessels going to the injured part,
thus minimizing any potential blood loss from the injured part.

Input from the pain nerves also excites both the main alpha
motor and the fusimotor nerves. This has the effect of 'splinting'
the injured part. When, for instance, we sprain a wrist, the
muscles moving that wrist are not continuously in spasm in
order to protect it from any movement that may further irritate
the injured part. Some movement is possible if done with care,
but any sudden inadvertent movement that further stimulates
the pain nerves provokes reflex muscle contraction. This
immediately splints the joint, protecting it from further hurt. In
our necks and backs the muscles are more easily fired off by an
input from the pain nerves. These muscles are not under such
good conscious control. In the spine there are lots of joints, all
with their own nerve supply, packed together. These joints are
behind us: we are not so aware what each individual joint is
doing. So when some part of our back is injured it is less easy
to protect the injured part. It is virtually impossible to protect
these joints from inadvertent movement, except possibly when
lying down, the muscles being so easily provoked into spasm.
If in fact there is some injury to the back it is therefore wise to
lie down immediately and stay there.

We have seen how the input from the pain nerves, particularly
the slow pain nerves, can be modified on its way up to the
brain. This modification is possible at the junctions between each

separate nerve, where neurotransmitters are responsible for the transference of the message from one nerve to the next. The modification possible is either an enhancement or an inhibition of the message. The chemical neurotransmitters can be modified by other neurotransmitters released when other nearby nerves are fired off, thus blocking or enhancing the link between one pain nerve and the next. The neurotransmitters released by the pain nerves can also be altered by chemical substances that have got there via the blood stream.

As a general rule stimulation of the larger-fibred sensing nerves in the body tends to block the input through the smaller pain nerves. It is therefore possible to reduce pain by stimulating these larger nerves. This can be done by stroking or gentle massage. The larger-fibred sensing nerves can also be stimulated by an electric current of the right wavelength and strength.

Machines capable of producing such a current are available on the market. They are called TENS machines (Transcutaneous Electrical Nerve Stimulation). If the terminals attached to these machines are placed on the skin near or at the source of pain and current is passed for a period of time, usually about twenty minutes, often there is a marked reduction of that pain. TENS is nearly if not as effective as acupuncture.

Movement, as long as it is not acutely painful, also stimulates larger sensing nerves, particularly the muscle spindle nerves and the larger sensing nerves round the joints. This is why pain is often less when we are on the move.

After a night's sleep our aching necks and backs tend to be stiffer and more sore. When asleep the input through the larger sensing nerves is at a minimum. It is only after moving around, stimulating these larger nerves, that we feel less pain and stiffness. Earlier generations used to be well aware of the value of movement in reducing aches and pains – hence the once popular rocking chair. They knew they could rock their pains away.

Pain input may also be modified by activity in other nerves in the brain itself, or by nerve fibres travelling down the spinal cord from the brain, or by chemicals produced elsewhere which can alter the neurotransmitters, reaching them via the blood stream. Pain is modified by how we feel and by what we are doing at any particular time. For instance, soldiers injured in the heat of battle may suffer horrific injuries without being aware of undue pain. Pain comes on when they are back at base hospital, away from danger.

If we are depressed or anxious pain is worse. If we are distracted and excited pain seems less. A state of panic, acute fear, hysteria, a dose of the screaming ab dabs, call it what you will, may aggravate the sense of pain out of all proportion to the input coming through the pain fibres. Pain is very subjective and is really an emotional response to the input through the pain nerves. This emotional response may be modified by previous learned conditioning in early childhood. Some people seem to feel pain more than others. There is a wide variation in individual responses to pain.

Some of us use pain in order to manipulate our environment: to seek increased sympathy from others, or to get out of impossible personal problems.

A few suffer from what could be described as the Martyr's Syndrome: 'I still manage to struggle on in spite of my terrible sufferings.'

Opiates – morphine and the likes – are known to be among the most effective painkillers. It is now known the body is capable of producing its own opiate-like substances. These are produced by some of the nerve cells and are capable of blocking the neurotransmitters responsible for the transference of messages between one pain nerve fibre and the next. Because they block pain they also indirectly reduce the excitability of muscle, and thus impart a feeling of relaxation and well-being. Sensing nerves which are stimulated may release these substances from offshoots which make contact with the pain nerve endings in the spinal cord, thus having a very local effect. If the stimulus is sufficient they may also be released into the blood stream from certain of the nerve cells in the brain, thus also having a more general effect.

It is thought that acupuncture may relieve pain because it stimulates the production of these body opiates, called endorphins. Certainly this would seem to be so in rabbits. Then again, there is a wide gulf between the habits of rabbits and humans.

Certain brain cells may also be stimulated to produce endorphins by an act of faith: 'I will feel better by taking these pills the doctor gave me because she emphatically stated I would.' This is known as the placebo response to medication.

Placebo effect

If a doctor sits on one side of the desk and the patient on the other, and (s)he hands that patient a prescription for medicine, even if that medicine contains nothing but sugar and water, about thirty per cent of patients will feel that it has done them some good. The harder the sell the stronger the effect. It is not that these thirty per cent of patients imagine they are better — they are *in fact* better. The act of faith in the doctor's ability to solve our problem stimulates our body to produce its own medicine: endorphins and possibly other as yet unknown chemicals.

If the doctor crosses to the other side of the desk and pulls and pushes the patient around and then says that this will make him or her better, approximately sixty per cent of hims and hers will in fact feel better. This is what is known as the enhanced placebo effect. Healers of all sorts over the ages have utilized this effect without being aware of what they were doing. The more ritual involved in the treatment the more effective it would seem to be. Witch doctors can be very effective.

In this era of scientific medicine any new treatment is subjected to the rigours of a clinical trial before it is recommended for use on patients. The most rigorous and objective type of trial is known as a double blind trial. It is not that the doctor and the patient have to be blind, but that neither of them have to know if the treatment handed out is what is supposed to be effective or is just a dummy treatment. A considerably higher proportion than thirty per cent of those receiving the effective treatment have to feel better before such treatment will be thought to be effective. When testing a physical treatment such as acupuncture this percentage has to be significantly over sixty per cent. So far this has not turned out to be so.

Then again, a sixty per cent or so cure rate is not a bad batting average for any treatment.

These trials can create a dilemma for the doctor. If one is using a form of treatment in which there is great faith, and if it seems to help patients who have not been helped by other forms of treatment, that great faith is probably contributing to its effectiveness. If the doctor then finds that such treatment is not significantly more effective than an enhanced placebo response what is he to do?

He may choose to ignore the facts and refuse to read the scientific journals and feel he knows best and just carry on. He may accept the facts and still carry on. He is then likely to have guilt feelings and will not sell his treatment so effectively, thus being less effective as a doctor. Or he may choose to abandon this form of treatment. If he does, others more ignorant or with less scruples will step in. From the patient's point of view, particularly if there is nothing better to offer, he or she may be better off and have a better chance of receiving help from the hard-selling ignorant con artist.

There we are! Seeking knowledge may be a painful process, and ignorance may be bliss, in more ways than one.

So far, the only parts of the anatomy of the spine we have not covered are the veins and arteries taking blood to and from the joints and muscles. These may be of importance to the orthopaedic or neurosurgeon but are of little importance to the average neck and back pain sufferer.

The Ravages of Age

If you are unfortunate enough to have pains in your neck or back in ninety-nine cases out of a hundred nothing will be found wrong with your spine which could not be accounted for by the normal ageing process.

If you have pain it may be called all sorts of things. For instance, starting from the neck down it may be labelled as: tension headache, occipital neuralgia, acute wry neck, cervical neuralgia, brachial neuralgia, cervical spondylosis, fibrositis, lumbago, arthritis, sciatica, and so on.

Do not let these names fool you into thinking they have much meaning as to what is really wrong. Most of them merely describe where you feel the pain of which you are only too well aware. These descriptive terms convey nothing about what is really causing the pain and are often used to satisfy the sufferer's need for a label and to hide the ignorance of those using the terms.

Ageing is really a wear-and-tear/repair process which is going on all the time, until there is less wear and tear that can be repaired. The chondrocytes gradually lose their ability to replace aged proteoglycans. Any repair to the worn or damaged ligaments and cartilage is done by fibrous scar tissue. This is less elastic than the original and thus the joints gradually stiffen up, and lose their range of movement. To protect the joints from excessive movement which may cause further damage, bone is laid down at the margin of the joints of both the discs and facets. The opposing cartilage in the facet joints becomes eroded and thinner. The bone beneath the cartilage hardens, thus helping it to cope with the increased stress due to loss of cushioning.

There is thus a gradual stiffening, and loss of range of motion in our spines.

Ageing as such need not be a painful process. The incidence of attacks of back pain in the community gradually reaches a peak at about the age of thirty-five. The incidence then starts to diminish after the age of fifty-five. This probably means some wear and tear has to take place before our backs become vulnerable to stress. After we reach the age of fifty-five we tend to become less active, and therefore less likely to overstress our backs. Either that or senior citizens have realized the futility of complaining.

In the low back the ageing process first becomes evident in the centre of the disc, the nucleus. Gradually the jelly-like centre is replaced by granular fibrous tissue. Starting with the inner rings of the annulus and slowly working out, the elastic collagen material is gradually replaced by non-elastic fibrous tissue. It is to be remembered the young healthy disc can withstand tremendous stress without coming to any apparent harm. This fibrous change in the annulus rings makes it more vulnerable to damage under stress. Such damage is usually first evident as tears of these inner rings.

When we move our backs the pivot of that movement is the centre of the disc, the nucleus. Therefore one would expect twisting and bending strains would place maximum stress at the greatest distance from this pivot point, the *outer* rings of the annulus. That the inner rings give out first is evidence they become weakened first, but not by stress.

The likely cause of this ageing process starting in the centre of the disc is simply the lack of adequate nourishment of the cells manufacturing replacement cartilage, the chondrocytes. Those in the centre of the disc are the ones most likely to be starved, hence the reason for ageing to start here.

What all this information boils down to is very simple: early ageing in our discs has nothing to do with the stresses we impose on our spines, but has everything to do with the fact that we are starving our chondrocytes. Simply, this means lack of movement.

There is evidence this premature ageing of our discs starts

very early in life. Remember, the centre of the disc contains no pain nerve endings. Considerable change can take place without any conscious awareness and by the time we get our first attack of back or neck pain a lot of wear and tear has taken place which cannot be altered.

Therefore to avoid premature ageing and thus the vulnerability of our discs to breakdown we must teach people — starting with the very young – how important movement is. No more long hours sitting in front of the goggle-box; wherever possible, walk instead of ride; frequent breaks in class for exercise, and so on.

By the time we reach the age of fifty or so the centre of our discs resembles sawdust and the sharp demarcation between the nucleus and annulus is lost. The proteoglycans, with their important ability to hold fluid, are lost, so the discs can no longer hold fluid under pressure, and quickly lose fluid when we sit. The less elastic fibrous tissue loses its compliance, so the discs become less able to absorb stress and there is a loss of mobility.

At this stage the disc does not rupture under stress as it could when we were younger. It is rare for the disc to rupture for the first time after the age of fifty-five.

In the upper part of the neck the changes of age are more apparent in the facet joints. This may be particularly so in the top two joints, leading to marked restriction of neck movements. It becomes difficult to see round to back one's car, and at the time of life when thoughts may stray to heaven, it becomes increasingly difficult to look there.

There is an artery supplying the base of the brain which runs in a bony canal just in front of the facet joints in the neck. This curls over the rim of the atlas to get to the hole in the base of the skull. Here it may get nipped, if the nearby joints are worn and thickened, when we look upwards for too long. It is therefore unwise to take on the task of painting the ceiling when we reach this age of stiffness. It is so easy to cause a temporary blocking of the blood supply to the base of the brain, which may cause sudden severe giddiness or a faint. This could lead to more serious damage due to the resulting fall off the ladder.

Problems with the disc

The prolapsed or ruptured disc

For a long time it has been known that the disc may rupture or prolapse. This is commonly called a 'slipped disc', though such a name gives a false idea of what has actually happened. In some discs the ageing process may become rapidly accelerated. The gelatinous nucleus may be converted into fibrous tissue which breaks into lumps (see Fig. 34). First the inner rings of the annulus give way, usually in concentric cracks. The nucleus gets squeezed between these cracks. This usually happens at the side of the back of the disc and usually affects discs normally subjected to most stress: the lower two in the low back.

When looked at from above these discs are slightly kidney-shaped. Repeated strains from bending forward tend to squeeze the disc nucleus backwards. The lobes of the kidney-shaped disc are more vulnerable to stress and the annulus is stronger at the

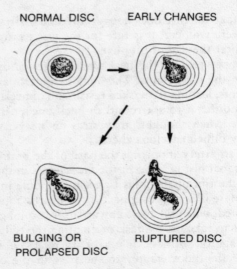

Figure 34 *The ruptured or prolapsed disc:* Cross section of a disc showing the changes which lead to rupture or prolapse.

front that at the back. Also, the long ligament running down the back of the disc tends to protect the middle of the back of the disc. Thus, the rings of annulus at each side of the back of the disc tend to give way first.

In time and with repeated bending stresses the damage reaches the outer rings of the annulus till the support is so weakened that the back of the disc bulges out. This is known as a disc hernia. The outer rings of the annulus may give way completely and bits of nucleus may be squeezed out, like toothpaste out of a tube. This is known as a disc rupture.

That this usually happens to the side of the back of the disc is important because the bulge or rupture is then close to where the nerve roots exit from the spine through the intervertebral foramen. Here space is limited and the bulge or rupture may trap the nerve root.

In time, if the outer rings are just weakened and bulging, a healing process takes place. The cartilage becomes fibrous and contracts down. The stretching of the outer rings irritates the margins of the vertebra where they are attached to the end plate cartilage. This stimulates the formation of new bone which juts out from the rim of the vertebra body. This acts as further protection to the weakened back wall of the disc.

This repair process takes time, measured in months rather than days.

While the disc is bulging out the pain nerves at the back of the disc will be continually irritated by the stretching, and thus there will be pain. As already mentioned, the centre of the disc contains no pain nerve endings and a lot of the early inner damage can take place without us being aware of what is happening. It is only when the outer rings of annulus break down that it becomes potentially painful.

When bits of nucleus and annulus rupture out into the spinal canal a chemical reaction to this invasion is provoked.

Part of our survival kit consists of a system whereby the body recognizes that something foreign is invading us. We have antibodies in our blood stream and tissues which are capable of attacking any foreign invader, or antigen. So that our own tissues are not attacked by our own antibodies there is a built-in recognition system which develops at a very early stage of our existence.

The inner disc contains substances not found in any other body tissue. These are shut off from the rest of the body. The disc has no blood supply and there is a membrane separating it from the rest of the body fluids which only allows certain substances to pass through.

Thus, it is thought the body has no recognition for its own inner disc material, and when the disc ruptures it is thought likely our own antibodies attack our own disc substance. This causes an acute local reaction with the consequent release of chemicals which irritate the pain nerve endings: a chemical or inflammatory reaction to injury causing chemical irritation of the pain nerve endings. This reaction involves the tissues surrounding the ruptured disc as it protrudes into the spinal canal, and in particular may involve the nerve roots leaving the spine. This may be very painful and is responsible for the more severe attacks of back pain and pain spreading down the legs.

If the extruded piece of disc material is small it may be completely eaten away by the antibody attack, and the break in the back wall of the disc heals up by the formation of fibrous scar tissue.

Some extrusions are quite large and when the invasion has been dealt with there still remains a lump of fibrous tissue. This no longer provokes an antibody reaction so the chemical pain stops, but the lump, which may become completely separated from the back wall of the disc, may still cause mechanical irritation of pain nerve endings.

The whole process of healing takes longer than a simple sprain, usually about two to three months. As a general rule, if pain goes on after this period of time it means that something else is the cause.

This particularly painful episode in life's journey has been described in detail because it is uppermost in most peoples' minds when they get back pain: 'Has my disc slipped?' Many minor episodes of disc rupture may happen without undue or prolonged pain. Post-mortem studies have revealed spinal canals containing many lumps of old extruded discs without there being a previous history of significant back pain.

Orthopaedic (bone and joint) surgeons vary in their enthusiasm for surgery when dealing with ruptured discs, but it is obvious that if a piece of disc has ruptured and is causing severe pain the only quick solution to the problem is the removal of the offending bit of disc. But it should be realized that surgery, though it usually relieves the immediate pain, does not cure or alter the worn disc which has caused the problem, and long-term studies suggest that having surgery does not reduce the chances of further episodes of back pain in the future.

In fact, ruptured discs are comparatively rare happenings. It has been estimated that only about one in every thousand attacks of back pain is considered severe enough to warrant the thought of an operation.

Diagnosing your own disc rupture

Occasionally this may be difficult, but it is often easy.

First, it does not necessarily require a severe strain to rupture the disc. The final straw that breaks the camel's back may be a quite trivial bending strain. The preceding changes weakening the inside of the disc may have been painless because of the lack of pain nerve endings inside the disc.

There may be a history of previous attacks of back pain before the final rupture. These previous attacks often have a tendency to become progressively more severe, last longer, and spread further down one leg with each attack.

When the outer rings of the annulus finally give way there will be an immediate stretching and distortion of the pain nerves in the back wall of the disc and in the outer lining, the dural sleeve, of the spinal cord. This will cause an immediate pain localized to the back. There may then be a lull of a few hours before the body's reaction to the extruded disc material becomes evident. Irritant chemicals produced by this reaction then cause a more severe chemical stimulation of the pain nerve endings. Such a reaction does not stop day or night so the pain is continuous – there is no complete let up. Getting off to sleep may be very difficult, requiring the help of pain killers. Sleep is usually disturbed by pain; and often the sufferer first wakes in pain only an hour or so after going to sleep. Getting back to sleep is difficult – it is often necessary to get up and move about for an hour or so before sleep is again possible. This movement is helpful because it stimulates the larger sensing nerves which help to block off the input from the pain nerves.

First thing in the morning is a particularly bad time. A lot of the larger sensing nerves capable of blocking the pain have not been at work while we have been resting, but the pain nerves have been continuously firing. It therefore takes at least an hour of gently moving about before the pain eases. It never lets up completely through the day and tends to get worse in the later afternoon. During the day, any continued activity aggravates the pain. Because of the associated increased pressure within the disc, sitting down for any length of time can be particularly painful.

The pain usually starts in the middle or across the low back. If the nerve roots coming out of the side of the spine become involved in the reaction to injury, as they frequently do, and if the piece of extruded disc presses or rubs against the roots, the pain will rapidly spread to the buttock, thigh, and leg. This is a severe pain spreading in a continuous line down the leg and often into the foot. The spread down the leg often starts in a matter of a few hours, at the most a day or so, after the start of the back pain. A vague pain spreading into the thigh and sometimes the calf a week or so after the onset of back pain is more likely to be a slight referred type of pain which may come from any part of the spinal joints or associated muscles.

It is not possible to examine oneself effectively, but examination by others may provide some pointers to the diagnosis. If someone gently raises your leg on the more painful side, with you keeping your knee straight, and if this suddenly aggravates the pain before an angle of 20 to 30 degrees elevation is reached, the diagnosis is probably a ruptured disc.

The sciatic nerve is formed from branches of the nerve roots in the low back. On its way down to the leg it travels behind the hip joint. When the straight leg is raised the hip acts as a pulley and stretch is therefore slowly applied to the nerve, till at about 20 degrees of elevation it begins to pull on the nerve roots in the hole at the side of the spine, the intervertebral foramen. This will further irritate the pain nerves there which are already irritated by the extruded lump of disc. This will aggravate the pain.

If pain is not produced until an angle of more than 30 degrees is reached, the pain is more likely being caused by sudden aggravation of painful muscle spasm. Even at less than 30 degrees, muscle spasm may still be the culprit.

As the nerve roots in the low back emerge from the spine, that part of the root containing the motor nerves which supply the muscles in the leg lies in front of the root. This means that if a lump of disc presses on the root from the front, as is most likely, it will be these motor nerve fibres which will be damaged.

If the motor nerve fibre is damaged it is no longer able to transmit messages, and the muscle supplied by the nerve fibre will no longer work. Also, the reflex connection between the muscle spindle stretch receptors and the associated muscle itself will be broken. In the low back the reflex connection most likely to be broken is that between the heel (achilles) tendon and the muscles in the calf. So that if someone taps this tendon with a rubber hammer there will no longer be a sudden twitch of the calf muscle — an ankle jerk.

If it is found your ankle jerk has gone there is no great cause for alarm. If the nerve fibre below the nerve cell is damaged, as long as the cell itself is still alive the fibre will regenerate again, though this will take months. If the reflex has gone the damage has been done, so there is no urgent need for surgery — the milk is already spilt. Also, the normal healing process will tend to shrink the piece of disc material so that it may no longer cause a nuisance to the nerve root.

If the nerve fibre is damaged, the muscle it supplies will no longer function properly. This means muscle weakness. This can be detected in the early stages, soon after the damage has been done, but not with a high degree of certainty. Muscles are tested by getting them to work against a resistance. For example, the muscle that moves the big toe upwards may be affected in a low back disc rupture. So someone presses on the top of your big toe with their thumb and asks you to push against that thumb as hard as you can. If the resulting pressure against the resisting thumb feels weaker on one side than the other it may suggest the motor nerve to that muscle is damaged. This is not a completely reliable test: when we are in pain the fear of provoking more pain makes us instinctively hold back when asked to move any part of our bodies even remotely related to the painful part.

If surgery is contemplated it may become necessary to identify the site and size of the ruptured disc. To do this accurately requires more complicated tests.

First, blood tests will provide no useful information. No currently available blood test will tell us that a disc has ruptured. They may help exclude other possible rare causes of similar sudden severe back and leg pain, but this is the limit of their usefulness.

Straight X-rays of the spine also provide little useful information. Millions of pounds are wasted each year on such examinations. X-rays outline the bones, not the soft tissues which includes the discs. At most, the X-ray may identify a disc which has been subjected to more wear and tear than its neighbours. The space between two adjacent vertebrae will be narrowed. But this does not necessarily mean this is the disc which has just ruptured and such a finding may lead the surgeon astray.

There are further specialized X-rays currently used. These involve the injection of dyes which are opaque to X-rays into the spinal canal. Such X-rays are reliable in identifying a ruptured disc if a dent in the dye can be seen, but not so reliable in excluding a ruptured disc if no dent can be seen. In a few patients they may cause unpleasant side effects, such as severe headaches.

The most reliable modern test available is the CAT scan (Computerized Axial Tomography). This is non-traumatic to the patient, involves no injections, is very reliable, but is traumatic to the pocket. It is expensive.

How to manage your own disc rupture, or have it managed by others, will be described in the chapters on treatment.

Disc problems in the neck

The discs in the neck rarely rupture but those in the lower neck may be subject to rapid ageing, leading to fibrous changes and narrowing of the discs. To protect the worn discs new bone is laid down at the rim of the vertebra bodies. These rims or bars jut out into the spinal canal, thus narrowing the available space for the spinal cord. More particularly, they may narrow the openings at the side, the intervertebral foramen. This may constrict the nerve roots. Bony spurs may form on the rims of the vertebra bodies which may irritate these nerve roots and provoke a reaction to injury.

Why such a condition should arise is not understood. In medical circles it is described as cervical spondylosis. It is more common amongst women, particularly those with a naturally marked curve in their neck. The ill effects of this process are most frequently felt in the middle years of life, the forties and fifties, whereas wear and tear in the upper neck is more likely to cause problems in the later years.

The bony spurs and thickening of the rims of the vertebral bodies can be seen on an ordinary X-ray, but if such changes show on your X-ray it does not necessarily mean they are causing problems. They are found just as frequently in those without problems as those with. In other words, as in the low back, the straight X-ray is usually a waste of time. Why these changes cause problems for some people but not for others is not clearly understood. The problems that do arise may follow a simple strain or overstress: lifting something up to a shelf above head level, or cleaning the windows, or painting the ceiling – in other words, working with the arms above shoulder height and with the head looking up. As we saw earlier, in the section on anatomy, such a position will narrow the spinal canal and the openings at the side where the nerve roots exit. If that opening is already constricted by a bony bar or spur of bone it may cause irritation of the nerve roots and set up a reaction to injury.

The pain caused by such a strain often starts at the back of the shoulder, then rapidly, within a few hours, spreads up the back of the neck, into the shoulder, and down the arm, often as far as the hand and even into some fingers and/or the thumb. As with nerve root pain in the low back this is severe and spreads in a continuous line down the arm.

How to cope with such a problem will be described in the chapters on treatment.

Disc problems in the thoracic (chest) spine

Problems with the discs in this part of the spine are surprisingly common; in fact so common as to be considered normal – which, of course, they are not. These problems were first described by a doctor from the Netherlands, whose name was Scheuermann. Since his published reports the problems have been described as Scheuermann's Disease.

Variations from what is considered to be normal tend to end up being labelled as this or that 'disease'. This establishes the problem as a medical problem. However, if that problem proves to be due just to excessive wear and tear, and once that wear and tear has taken place there is nothing which can be done to put the clock back, it really cannot be described as a disease. It may be preventable but certainly it is not treatable. This is so with Scheuermann's Disease.

Scheuermann's Disease This condition begins during early adolescence, usually at the time of an associated growth spurt, commonly between the ages of eleven to seventeen.

What happens is this. The end plate cartilage on the top and bottom of each vertebra body becomes weakened and cracks. This allows the jelly-like nucleus to be squeezed through the cracks. That part of the vertebral body where growth takes place lies just under the end plate. The growing cells are damaged by the extruded disc nucleus. Therefore the growth taking place just under the end plate is uneven, and as bone is laid down in the growing cells the top or lower surface of the vertebra body looks pitted. It shows up on an X-ray as an uneven line to the top or bottom edge of the vertebra body (see Fig. 35). This happens most frequently between the eighth thoracic (chest) vertebra and the first lumbar (low back) vertebra, with a peak of incidence at about the tenth thoracic vertebra.

Relating to the loss of disc nucleus there is premature ageing of the disc, which becomes stiff and narrowed. Because the damage to the growing cells happens more frequently towards the front of the vertebral body, growth is interfered with more at the front than the back. Therefore, as the body grows it tends to become more wedge shaped: higher at the back than the front. Thus, the end result can be an increase in the forward curve of this part of the spine which is stiffer than it should be.

You may well ask, 'So what? The part of the spine most

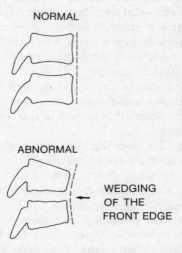

NORMAL

ABNORMAL

WEDGING
OF THE
FRONT EDGE

Figure 35 *Scheuermann's Disease, Side view of two thoracic (chest) vertebrae:* Damage to the end plate and the growing cells just under the end plate leads to irregular pitting of the two opposing surfaces of the vertebrae. These changes are more marked at the front of the vertebra. This causes a wedging of the front edge. The premature ageing of the disc results in a narrowing of the gap between each vertebra.

affected by these changes gives least trouble as we get older, so such changes should not matter very much.'

In fact, it does matter, though this is not as yet generally recognized. Recent research has shown that those who show evidence of having had this problem have more than double the chance of developing evidence of premature ageing in the low back joints. Why should this be so?

Recently, a small team, including the author, had a look at the local population of seventeen and eighteen year olds. We felt that more needed to be known about what causes Scheuermann's Disease. If there is to be hope of preventing premature breakdown in the low back, we need to know how to prevent Scheuermann's Disease.

Previous reports have suggested that heavy manual work during the vulnerable adolescent growth period may be responsible. Compression forces have to play a part in forcing the nucleus of the discs through the cracks in the end plates. A lot of the youngsters in the part of New Zealand I come from do get involved in quite heavy work, especially on the farms, and a lot play vigorous sport involving a lot of potentially harmful compression stresses.

We examined 500 of the seventeen and eighteen year olds in the local schools and teachers' training college. This was a statistically significant cross section of this age group still in the educational system.

Each one of these 500 filled in a questionnaire, to determine past work and sporting activities (which sports they had played, and for how long; what spare time holiday work and farm work they had done), and also to pinpoint those who had had previous back problems.

Their spines were examined, to look for clinical evidence of previous Scheuermann's Disease, and for evidence of other factors which may play a part in back problems, such as one leg being longer than the other.

Each one then had an X-ray of their spines. This was a single side-on view, concentrating on the mid and low dorsal and upper lumbar spine – the regions most often affected by Scheuermann's Disease. These X-rays were examined by an independent expert, who had no access to the questionnaire or examination results. The completed questionnaire, examination reports and X-ray reports were then handed to an independent expert statistician, who translated them into computerese.

These are the results which came out of the computer: 56 per cent of the males and 30 per cent of the females had X-ray evidence of Scheuermann's Disease in varying degrees of severity.

When we first started on this survey, taking into account previous reports, we expected to find an incidence of about 10 per cent – not nearly 60 per cent in males and 30 per cent in females. These are alarming figures.

A further alarming result was the high incidence of previous attacks of back pain amongst these youngsters: 60 per cent of the males and 52 per cent of the females had already suffered previous attacks of back pain which had lasted for one week or more. These attacks were significantly more common in males who had X-rays showing the changes of Scheuermann's Disease, but not in females.

An unexpected result: those who had been involved in heavy work or had taken part in particularly strenuous sports were no more prone to Scheuermann's Disease than the rest. The only activity which nearly reached significance level was rowing. Rowing, of course, is the only sport involving a lot of sitting. Another significant result: males who had been confined to bed because of illness or injury for two weeks or more at some stage between the ages of eleven and seventeen were significantly more prone to this problem. This confirms a long-held belief that bed can be a dangerous place, at least for us males.

So, what do these findings mean? They mean one thing and one thing only: youngsters' spines can cope with dynamic stresses imposed by heavy work or strenuous sports without coming to apparent harm.

If Scheuermann's Disease is looked at as simply being due to poor nourishment of our cartilage and disc chondrocytes, leading to faulty production of replacement disc and cartilage tissue the whole problem begins to make sense.

From what has already been said about the nourishment of

our chondrocytes it may be understood that such faulty nourishment will simply be due to lack of adequate movement. This means too much sitting on our behinds.

It may also mean too long lying on our beds.

We know that in the sitting position the pressure inside the disc is comparatively high, and that fluid tends to be squeezed out of the disc. We also know that when lying down the pressure is comparatively low and fluid is sucked into the disc.

But there is a limit to how much fluid may be sucked in or squeezed out. When that limit is reached there will be no movement of fluid. Due to the closely packed proteoglycan substance such movement is slow, and to cater for the nutritional needs of the chondrocytes requires frequent movement of the disc, to aid the diffusion of nutrients.

Before the disc substance is able to break through the cartilage end plate and thus disrupt the growing bone cells, this end plate has to be weakened. It would now seem clear that such weakening and cracking is not due to everyday trauma. This must mean such breakdown is due to the breakdown of cartilage weakened and not being adequately replaced by starved chondrocytes.

Then why does such damage mainly affect the lower dorsal spine, and why does it reach a peak of incidence at about the tenth dorsal level, falling away in incidence above and below this point?

The reason for this becomes clear if the following is taken into account. The chondrocytes will be equally affected by lack of movement in all parts of the spine. When sitting, movement is still taking place, most times, in the neck, shoulders, and thus the upper part of the dorsal (chest) spine. This movement becomes less the further down the spine one goes. So, the problem becomes evident in the low dorsal spine, and the rest of the spine should be equally affected. But the further down the spine one goes the stronger and thicker the discs become. Thus the damage becomes less evident, but nonetheless it must still be taking place. This explains why those who have evidence on their X-rays of Scheuermann's Disease also tend to suffer premature ageing in the lower spine at a later date. The stage has been set but it takes longer for the effects to be seen. In other words, the changes seen in the X-ray in the lower dorsal spine are just the thin edge of the wedge.

In practical terms what this means is very simple. It is necessary for all our educators and parents to have a rethink about how to rear our offspring. A pattern of living which includes more activity has to be programmed into the young computers, and such a pattern has to become part of our way of life throughout life. Movement need not be vigorous but it certainly needs to be frequent.

As with our hearts, teeth, and so on, we need to start looking after our spines at an early age.

Frequently, Scheuermann's Disease occurs without the knowledge of the sufferer: it can be silent. If it does hurt this is usually because of some added strain or minor injury. Usually no treatment is necessary, just a bit of rest. Some local treatment to associated tight muscles may give relief. More about this later, in the chapters on treatment.

Problems with the facet joints

The facet joints in our spines are subject to the same wear and tear process as similar synovial joints. With a few exceptions these include most of the rest of the body's joints.

As we get older there is a higher incidence of wear and tear changes in these spinal joints than in any other of the body's synovial joints. This implies that they are subject to more stress. In the low back, changes of ageing start in the middle of the disc. As these changes progress, more stress tends to fall on the facet joints. As the disc becomes narrower and the elastic disc material is gradually replaced by more fibrous, less elastic material, there is a loss of resilience and the ability to absorb impact and torsion stresses. The pattern of rocking over the nucleus is altered, and the stress tends to be transferred to the facet joints. This is particularly so at the bottom of the spine. Here, because of the alignment of the facet joints and the natural forward curve of the spine, the facet joints have to cope with increasing weight-bearing and shear stresses, to prevent the whole spine from slipping forward.

The ageing changes in the facet joints gradually restrict the range of motion allowed by the joint: we become stiffer. The capsules of the joints become tighter and less elastic. The muscles moving the joints adjust to the gradual loss of movement, protecting them from possible stressful movement. If, say, you move one of your fingers to its maximum range, and then take hold of that finger, you will then find you can push it a bit further than you could by moving it yourself. This is the safety margin which does not allow us to move our joints to the point where it may do them harm. As the joints get stiffer this safety margin is maintained. It is obviously regulated by a feed-back of information from the sensing nerves in the joint casing.

Ageing changes in the facet joints are progressive through life, therefore if these changes were responsible for a lot of our neck and back pains we would expect more trouble the older we get. This does not happen: attacks of back pain tend to get less in our later years. Mainly for this reason these joints have been somewhat neglected as a main source of problems.

Manipulation is a form of treatment which has stood the test of time. Most techniques of manipulation involve a sudden movement of the facet joints – 'popping' the joints. Manipulators have sought reasons for how this could help, and for what could be wrong with the facet joints which could be helped by such a manoeuvre. It has been suggested these joints may become jammed, like a partly shut drawer, or that fringes of the joint lining, the synovial lining, may get trapped between the two joint surfaces. In the neck and low back small menisci have been found. These are little tongues of cartilage coming from the inside of the joint casing. They help the joints absorb impact stresses and spread the load on the joints by increasing the contact area between the joint surfaces. They have the same function as knee cartilages. It has been suggested they may become trapped between the joint surfaces. Because they are supplied by pain nerve endings this could be a cause of sudden pain in the neck or low back.

No satisfactory evidence has in fact been found to show that any of these things do happen, at least with any degree of frequency. Post mortem examinations have shown these joints and surrounding ligaments have been subject to previous sprains or tears, but such happenings could not in any conceivable way be helped by manipulation. In fact, vigorous movement imposed on healing tissue would tend to do harm rather than good.

The whys and wherefores of manipulation will be described in the treatment chapters. Suffice to say it probably helps by stimulating the sensing nerves in the facet joint casings, which has the effect of reflexly relaxing associated tight, painful muscles.

Thus far, the main hazards to our ageing facet joints are simple sprains and strains. Rarely, if the injuring force is great enough, small bone fractures may happen round the joints. These may account for prolonged pain, until the fracture heals.

Problems with the muscles

With advancing years, not all that advanced in some, all of us develop small tender areas within our muscles. These areas may not cause any problems and we are only aware of their existence if someone gives the muscle a good poke, but under certain circumstances they may become a source of pain. In fact, they are probably the most common source of on-going pain in our framework.

Nowadays, such areas are known as trigger points.

Trigger points

Exactly what trigger points are is still a subject of some controversy, but there is no doubt they exist. Locating them is a learned skill. Once that skill has been acquired there can be no doubt about their existence. As a general rule, the more you look for them the more you will find.

Trigger points are small areas within a muscle which are very tender when that area of the muscle is prodded. They feel like a small knot or small band within the muscle.

They occur in approximately the same place within the same muscle in different individuals. This means if you know where to look for them in one person you will know where to look in everyone else. The reason for this is not clear, but there must be a reason.

Most of our trigger points are described as latent, which means they are not causing any symptoms, but they may become active (hot) and cause pain. If they become active they have what is called a positive 'jump' sign: when you press on them the sufferer jumps, and the muscle can be seen to twitch. When active or 'hot', trigger points are capable of causing local or referred pain and a feeling of numbness or pins and needles. The sites of the local and referred pain have characteristic patterns for each individual muscle. This means if you are aware of pain in a particular region you should be able to tell which particular muscle trigger point is responsible.

Let's take some examples. Trigger points in the muscles which move the shoulder, round the back of the shoulder blade, may cause vague ill-defined pain in the upper arm and forearm, and occasionally pins and needles or numbness in the hand and some or all of the fingers and thumb. The site of the pain in the arm depends on which muscle contains the trigger point.

A trigger point in the muscles at the back of the neck, just below the skull, may cause a headache, felt at the back of the head and sometimes spreading through to behind the eyes.

A trigger point in the muscles to the side of the spine at the level of the junction between the chest and low back part of the spine may cause pain felt in the low back.

A trigger point in the rump muscles may cause pain spreading down the thigh and even into the leg.

A trigger point in the back of the calf muscle may cause pain in the heel.

Many more examples could be given. Charts showing the spread of pain from different trigger points are available (see Fig. 36). Those responsible for looking after others' aches and pains have, or should have them.

A latent trigger point may be converted into a hot one by several events, such as excessive use of the muscle, sitting in a cold draught, getting chilled, getting uptight, or by a neck or back strain.

They are most common in the back and neck muscles moving the spine, and in the more central muscles which move the shoulders and hips.

When a muscle becomes 'hot', pain nerve endings are being fired off within it. This probably means the trigger point consists

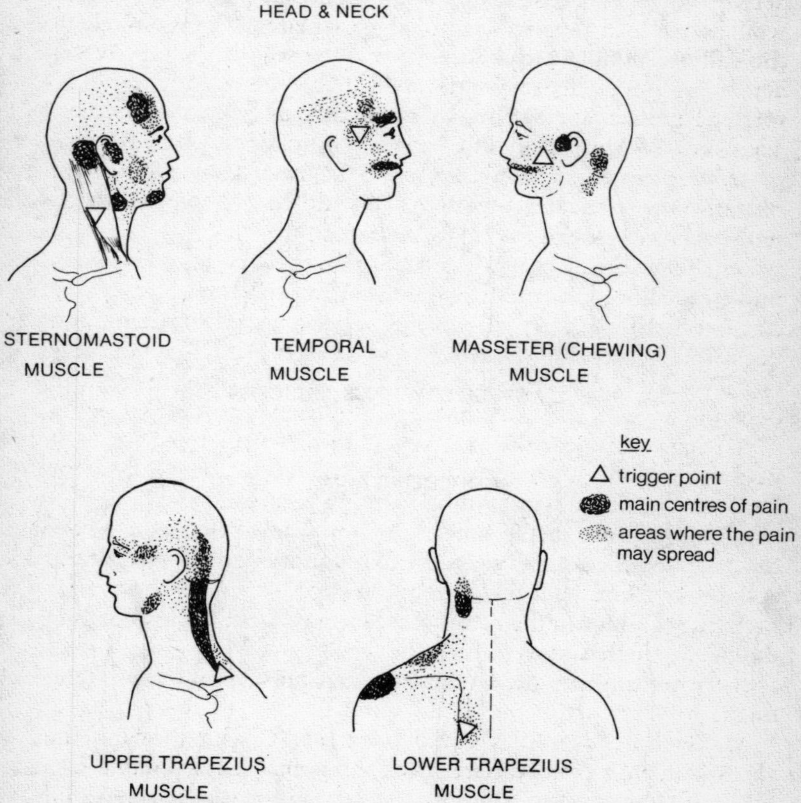

HEAD & NECK

STERNOMASTOID
MUSCLE

TEMPORAL
MUSCLE

MASSETER (CHEWING)
MUSCLE

key
△ trigger point
● main centres of pain
⬚ areas where the pain may spread

UPPER TRAPEZIUS
MUSCLE

LOWER TRAPEZIUS
MUSCLE

Figure 36 *Common sites of trigger points and where they hurt*

CHEST & BACK

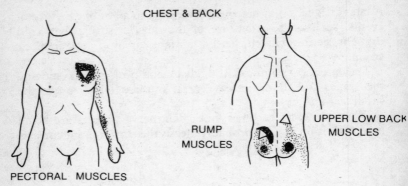

PECTORAL MUSCLES

RUMP
MUSCLES

UPPER LOW BACK
MUSCLES

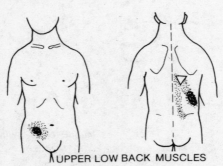

UPPER LOW BACK MUSCLES

SHOULDER & ARM

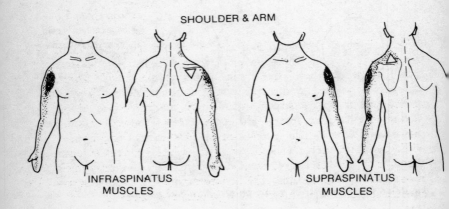

INFRASPINATUS
MUSCLES

SUPRASPINATUS
MUSCLES

LOWER EXTREMITY

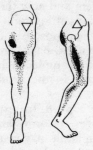

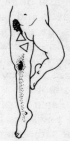

RUMP MUSCLES   ADDUCTOR MUSCLES

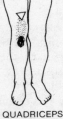

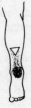

QUADRICEPS
MUSCLES   CALF MUSCLES

of muscle fibres that are contracted down, in spasm, and will not relax. This will distort the pain nerve endings. Such spasms will also interfere with the blood supply to the muscle fibres. The energy burned by the constantly active muscle will lead to accumulation of wastes from this burning, and these wastes will also irritate the pain nerves. The stage is thus set for an ongoing vicious circle of muscle spasm—pain—further muscle spasm.

To maintain such a vicious circle will require a further input through the muscle nerves from elsewhere. This further input is most likely to be through the fusimotor nerves, supplying the muscle spindles. Let's have a look at why this happens.

It has already been explained how these fusimotor nerves are part of our arousal or alerting system and how they are responsible for our neck and back muscles getting tight when we get uptight. These are the muscles which most frequently contain trigger points. In other words, the neck, back, and other more central muscle groups behind us are not under such good central control and are thus more sensitive to the primitive alerting nerves, the fusimotors.

When stimulated by a poke or a prod, in response to that stimulation a newborn baby moves its arms and legs in all directions. The same stimulus to an adult may result in a return poke in the eye. The transition between these two responses is due to a complex learning process of muscle control. Instead of haphazardly firing off, our muscles come under increasing central, brain, control, so that just the necessary ones are fired in order to produce a controlled response to the stimulus. Such control is due to a process called selective inhibition. This means we learn to suppress all the motor nerves not necessary for achieving the desired movement.

Thus, gradually our muscles come under increasing central control to the extent that under normal conditions, whatever exciting or inhibiting influences are coming in to the motor nerve at the spinal cord level from other sensing nerves, they do not fire off without a central command so to do.

The central computer in the brain has taken full command of our motor responses to any stimulus. Even when we are threatened and the alerting system is on red alert we can still respond in a purposeful way to the threat. The input through the fusimotor nerves will excite the motor nerves and thus make them more sensitive, speeding their response to the central command, but that central control still remains.

The ability to control muscle action varies from individual to individual. Some are better co-ordinated than others. Research has indicated that the less well co-ordinated are more prone to chronic neck and back problems. It is also recognized that individuals under increased emotional stress are much more prone to developing sore necks and backs.

There is no doubt central control is more highly developed in our limb muscles, particularly in those moving our fingers. Using so-called bio-feedback techniques individuals can learn to fire off just one single motor nerve, suppressing all others. It is also possible to learn to relax a muscle completely, totally inhibiting motor nerve activity. This is relatively easy with those muscles moving the hand and foot, but the nearer to the back and neck one gets the more difficult it becomes. With the muscles in the back of the neck and spine it is very difficult, in some individuals impossible.

This is why these bio-feedback techniques have not proved to be a sure fire success in teaching individuals to relax their own neck and back muscles. The fusimotor system is still able to keep them uptight. Such an influence will help to maintain the pain—muscle spasm—pain cycle within the trigger point.

Increased fusimotor nerve activity may be caused by overactivity in our alerting system: we are anxious, frightened, angry, over-stressed, uptight, call it what you will.

This increased activity may also have a local cause. As we get older so do our joints, particularly those in our spines. Use of these worn joints will cause increased activity in the sensing nerves within the joint casing, particularly the Type 1 tension-measuring nerves. These seem capable of exciting the fusimotor nerves supplying related muscles.

If we overstress some part of our neck or back there is often first a local pain. Sometimes, after a few days or a week or so, the pain may spread from the neck to the shoulder, and later down the arm; or from the low back to the rump, and later down the leg. At this stage examination will reveal the presence of hot trigger points in the related muscles. Remember, most muscles have a nerve supply coming from at least two adjacent segmental levels of the spinal cord. The muscles developing the trigger points have at least some of their nerve supply coming from the same segmental level supplying the spinal joint which has been overstressed. If the original joint strain has healed, any reaction to the injury, healing, is over and done with, though the pain that has developed from the trigger points may persist.

At this stage, local treatment to the trigger points will give relief, but if, for instance, the joint injury is more severe and the reaction to this injury is still going on, it does not matter what you do to the trigger points – they will not go away.

Manipulation will be described in greater detail later. Probably its main, if not only, effect is reflexly to relax uptight muscle. This may be by the stimulation of sensing nerves round the joints which are capable of inhibiting, dampening down, the fusimotor nerves supplying the associated muscles, or it may be by blocking sensing nerves which are already overstimulating the associated fusimotor nerves.

If the original joint strain has settled and if you then have this joint manipulated, the very tender trigger points will immediately stop being tender and the pain will go away. If the owner of the hot trigger points is very uptight and remains so it does not matter what is done to the joints or the trigger points – they will still keep on hurting.

From everything we have discussed here, you will see how important is disorganized nerve activity, probably mainly the fusimotor nerves, in the production and perpetuation of these potentially painful trigger points.

Attempts to find out exactly what trigger points are have been made. Pieces of muscle taken from the sites of trigger points (muscle biopsy) have been looked at under the microscope. These examinations have only demonstrated normal muscle. In some long-standing trigger points changes have been found which are consistent with a long-standing lack of oxygen, but that is all.

Trigger points occupy only a small area in the muscle and it is possible the exact trigger point has not yet been examined, but it seems likely that in fact trigger points are normal (physiological) and not abnormal (pathological) states within the muscle. This fits in with the fact that even if a trigger point has been giving trouble for years it will disappear with treatment just as quickly as one of recent onset, at least for a time.

When a muscle fibre contracts it creates an electric potential. This can be recorded by special machines, called EMG's (Electro-Myelographic). Attempts to record increased electrical activity in these trigger points have largely failed. But this would be expected if the increased activity was in the fusimotor nerves, since minute contractions of the spindle muscle fibres are not detectable by EMG's. The increased activity in the main muscle fibre would only be apparent when the trigger point was stimulated by the slightest stretch: when the muscle is prodded such a small stretch would result.

Trigger points may be treated successfully in several different ways. Each method has its own following of enthusiasts. Probably, they are all equally effective and sometimes ineffective.

Simple pressuring of the trigger point is probably as effective a method of pain relief as any. This is important for the reader to know: it is something which can be done at home. A lot of trigger points are difficult to get at by oneself, so help will be needed. This may come from one's nearest and dearest.

All that is required is a thumb, sometimes an elbow, or some suitable blunt weapon. Really firm pressure (see Fig. 37) is applied to the skin overlying the trigger point. This hurts. Some partners are reluctant to cause discomfort to their loved ones,

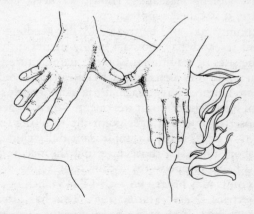

Figure 37 *How to pressure a trigger point:* Keep a firm pressure on the very sore spot until it stops hurting – usually two to three minutes. If it takes longer than this, simple pressure will probably not help.

others thrive on it. It is important to understand this pressure has to be maintained until the pain stops. With a really 'hot' trigger point this usually takes about three minutes. As the pain decreases the small hard knot of muscle can be felt to slowly melt away, if the thumb has not become too numb to feel anything. This pressuring can be done on a daily basis. As the original pain becomes less it will be found that pressuring becomes less painful and the knot of muscle will take less time to melt.

If the trigger point is unbearably tender, and if after three minutes there is no lessening of the pain, or the knot of muscle shows no sign of melting, local treatment should be abandoned. If this is the situation it means there is something outside the trigger point which is keeping it 'hot'. This may be a reaction to injury in the associated joints which is still going on, inflammation in the joints, or it may be the owner of the trigger point has too much activity in his or her alerting system, is too uptight.

Pressuring has been known to be an effective treatment for trigger points for a long time. At the turn of the century German doctors called such treatment 'Gelotripsie'. Simply translated this means 'violent massage'. Today, to keep upsides with acupuncture, it is called acupressure.

Trigger points may also be treated by dry needling: acupuncture. Recent research has shown a highly significant co-relation between the sites of traditional Chinese acupuncture points and the trigger point sites determined by Western medicine. Thus two separate cultures have reached the same conclusion about the value of local trigger point treatment. When an acupuncture needle is inserted into a trigger point the resulting sensation is described as 'Che'. This is an unpleasant dull aching sensation lasting a short time. To those inserting the needle it feels as though it is being gripped – by locally contracting muscle.

Trigger points may be treated with TENS machines (Transcutaneous Electrical Nerve Stimulation). This has already (page 65) been described. It seems to be as effective as acupuncture, and yet probably works, or does not work, by different mechanisms. They both take longer than pressuring – twenty minutes as against three minutes – but they are less painful. Perhaps this is why they take longer.

Many doctors inject trigger points with a weak solution of a local anaesthetic. This works by deadening the pain nerves, thus breaking the pain—muscle spasm—pain cycle. Some doctors add steroids to the injections. These steroids are powerful anti-inflammation agents. But there is no inflammation so their use is illogical.

One of the latest fashions is to spray the muscle containing the trigger point from end to end with a cold spray. These special cold sprays are used extensively in dealing with minor sports injuries. The method is as follows: holding the spray about 50 cm away from the skin, the muscle is sprayed over its whole length, from origin to insertion. At the same time the sprayer gently stretches the relaxed muscle. The stretching irons out the offending trigger point.

Enthusiasts for such treatment have observed that if the skin over the muscle is cooled too much the muscle will not stretch out. The reason for this is obvious. A cooling breeze sooths the furrowed brow – light cooling of the skin is pleasant. It relaxes uptight muscle. On the other hand, a cold wind makes us shiver and shake. Gentle cooling stimulates sensing nerves in the skin which reflexly inhibit muscle nerves, whilst chilling stimulates sensing nerves which have the opposite effect.

In summary, you, and possibly someone else, can manage to deal with your own painful trigger points. You may need to be shown where they are but from there on you can cope. Pressuring is simple, quick, but tolerably painful. You could use a TENS machine – they are available on the market – but you would need to be shown how. Other treatments require medical or para-medical assistance.

SECTION 3
Attacks of Pain

Likely trouble spots: how they are strained, and where they hurt

If you've read this far, you are in a pretty good position to take stock of the situation if you are unfortunate enough to be smitten by neck or back pain.

The parts of the spine most likely to give trouble are those which are subject to the most wear and tear. Starting at the bottom and working up, these are: *The lowest two joints*. They have to carry the heaviest load. The low back curve makes these joints subject to a lot of shear stress. They are protected from this by strong bracing ligaments. The tail piece (sacrum) is joined to the pelvic bones by two strong semi-rigid joints, the sacro-iliac joints. The pelvis is a fairly rigid structure whilst the spine is mobile. Maximum stress falls on the junction between the mobile and the rigid — one gives, the other does not — thus the maximum stress falls on these bottom two joints.

The sort of strains likely to damage these joints are those involving bending forward and twisting at the same time. This imposes increased pressure and stress on the back wall of the disc. If this is already badly worn it may rupture. Excessive stresses may also fall on the discs, if you have a heavy fall on your behind. A bending, twisting strain also imposes maximum stress on the ligaments and facet joint casings which lie behind the pivot point of bending.

Pain from these lowest joints usually starts in or across the low back, and may remain there. It may also spread into the groin, buttock, various regions of the thigh and leg, and even into the foot and toes. If it spreads, look for 'hot' trigger points, especially in the rump muscles.

The next joints up almost if not as likely to be overstressed are those *at the junction between the chest (thoracic) part of the spine and the first of the low back joints*. Remember, here there is a sudden change in the alignment of the facet joints: the facet joints in the thoracic spine allow twisting but those in the low back do not. In the chest region twisting is restricted by the attachment of a fairly rigid rib cage, but the lowest two ribs are short and do not have such a rigid attachment: they do not restrict twisting quite so much. Again, maximum stress tends to fall on the junction between the mobile and the rigid, thus twisting stresses may easily overstress the lowest two chest vertebrae. Also remember, these joints may have already suffered previous wear and tear from Scheuermann's Disease, thus being a bit more worn than the rest.

A twisting stress with the back more or less straight will thus tend to overstress this region of the spine rather than the low back.

Pain from this part of the spine may be felt in the upper part of the low back, but also it may only be experienced in the low back. It may spread into the loin and lower stomach (you may think you have a kidney stone or an appendix) and into the upper part of the rump.

One of the strange things about pain, particularly if coming from one of these low back joints, is as follows: if you strain one of the joints in the low back, causing pain for some time, and then strain another joint at a later period, the pain from the second strain, although coming from a different joint, is often experienced in the same place as during the first attack.

Again, if the pain spreads look for trigger points. These may be found in the muscles just to the side of the spine, approximately level with the strained joint. Another common site is just above the brim of the pelvis at the back.

Moving up the spine, the next likely trouble spot is in *the middle of the chest (thoracic) part of the spine*. This is at the apex of the backward curve in this part of the spine. (Engineers will tell you the apex, middle, of a curve is subject to more stress than the rest). Often the joints below this level are stiff because of previous Scheuermann's Disease, and mobile joints next to stiff ones can be more easily strained. These joints may be over-stressed by a bending—lifting strain, or by reaching up to put something on a high shelf. Often they are overstressed just by prolonged sitting, bent over a flat-topped desk or a car steering wheel.

Pain from these overstressed joints may be isolated to the middle of this part of the back. Sometimes it may spread round the chest wall to the front of the chest. This may lead you, and your doctor, to think you have pleurisy.

If the pain spreads round the chest, trigger points will be found in the muscles at the side of the spine, level with the strained joint, and also often in the small muscles between each rib.

Moving further up, the next likely trouble area is in *the lowest two neck joints*. As already mentioned, the discs in the lower part of the neck are prone to early wear and tear. The upper part of the thoracic spine is held fairly rigid by the upper part of the rib cage. There is very little movement here but plenty in the neck. Again, maximum stress falls on the mobile part at the junction with the immobile.

Pain from these overstressed joints may remain at the base of the neck. It often spreads to behind the shoulder and then down the arm. Remember, the muscles which move the shoulder get their nerve supply from the neck, so if the pain spreads trigger points will be found in these muscles.

The very mobile *mid part of the neck* is particularly prone to stress, usually the second to the fourth joints down. This is particularly so in the so-called 'whiplash' injury, which commonly happens when one's car is hit from behind. The car and one's body is suddenly pushed forward but the free head stays behind: thus the neck is suddenly jerked backwards. If the head is jerked forwards the chin hits the chest, and this stops the neck from bending too far. When the neck is jerked backwards there is no such protection and the joints are more easily overstressed.

There are varying degrees of severity in such injuries. Fortunately, most of them are minor and there is just a general overstressing of the joints and supporting ligaments. Remember, the pivot point of any bending is the disc nucleus. Therefore, any sudden jerk backwards will lead to a stretch of the ligament in front of the pivot point, the broad strong anterior (front) longitudinal ligament. With severe injuries this may be torn. This leads to local bleeding and a small pool of blood may collect in front of the spine leading to a feeling of fullness in the throat and difficulty in swallowing. An even more severe injury may force the facet joints, behind the pivot point, into each other, causing them to fracture. This damage can be seen on an X-ray. An even more severe injury may crush the back of the bodies of the vertebrae into each other, causing a crush fracture. This type of injury will also be seen on an X-ray.

Fortunately, nearly all whiplash injuries are minor and an X-ray shows no evidence of injury.

It was hoped the more widespread use of car head rests would reduce the incidence of whiplash injuries. According to one report, this is not so. Therefore, there is more to this type of injury than meets the eye.

Such minor injuries lead to a pain in the back of the neck, often starting a few hours or the next day after the accident. This may spread down to the shoulders and up into the head, leading to headaches in the back of the head and sometimes through to behind the eyes. Such pain has the bad habit of keeping on keeping on. If there has been some minor ligament damage this should heal up in two weeks or so and that should be that – the pain should stop. But often it does not.

Because it has been the result of a known accident such an ongoing problem often ends up in the hands of lawyers and orthopaedic (bone and joint) specialists. Due to the lack of objective evidence of injury the latter become frustrated and they both prosper. Some orthopaedic specialists deny there is such a thing as a whiplash injury. It is a figment, they argue, of the imagination of the sufferer, a compensation neurosis. But it is not. It is more complicated, and what seems to happen is this. Injury to one's car has a special significance to most of us. It is a deep personal insult and a sudden threat to our sense of security. This triggers off fear, anxiety, anger, which leads to increased activity in our alerting system. The minor injury to the neck joints provokes reflex local muscle spasm. This activates local latent trigger points which become the source of ongoing pain. Attempts at local treatment to the overstressed neck joints and local trigger points fails to give relief because of the general increased activity in the fusimotor nerves. Lack of improvement creates more anxiety. Anxieties about the cost of car repairs, possible litigation, also help to perpetuate the problem. So, the vicious circle of pain—muscle spasm—further pain goes on.

The top two joints of the neck tend to show increased wear and tear as we get older. This limits our view of heaven and the ability to see behind us when backing the car. These joints are prone to strain with blows to the head. This happens frequently to boxers and soccer players, when heading the ball. Remember, the first neck vertebra, the atlas, allows free nodding of the head backwards and forwards, but the second one, the axis, does not. Thus, if the head is suddenly snapped back this is where the stress will fall.

Strains to these joints may lead to severe headaches in various parts of the head and face. When someone is knocked out or concussed the resulting so-called post-concussion headache often results from overstress of these joints.

The headaches may be associated with other odd symptoms, such as a feeling of unsteadiness, a muzziness in the head, or fuzziness of vision – you may end up with several pairs of glasses, none of which are much help. There is a condition which has been labelled as 'soccer players' migraine' which has its origin in the overstressing of these joints.

The overloaded coping system syndrome

Some of us may have the misfortune to develop a pain in our back or neck or both, which just keeps on for no apparent reason. This may follow some relatively minor strain such as a whiplash injury, or it may start for no apparent reason. Instead of going away in the usual two weeks or so it just keeps on keeping on. Help is sought from doctors, physiotherapists, chiropractors, acupuncturists, and so on. No one is able to give more than very short lasting relief. In fact, sometimes the offered treatment may seem to make the pain worse, at least for a time.

A careful examination reveals a lot of hot trigger points, at least four. These are more common in the muscles at the side of the spine and are concentrated in the area where the pain is felt. If someone presses firmly on the spine several of the spine joints feel more tender than they should. Sometimes the pain spreads to other joints in the arms and legs. These may be tender and nearby muscles may contain hot trigger points.

It is not a generally recognized problem. A lot of doctors are not even aware of its existence. It has been labelled as 'Primary Fibromyalgia' or the 'Acute Fibrositis Syndrome'. Many sufferers of so-called ME (Myelo-Encephalomyelitis) do in fact have this problem. These names convey the vision of a disease which needs a cure. In desperation some sufferers end up being labelled as neurotic, implying the sufferer is abnormal and his or her imagination is at fault. This is unfair and not true. It is not a disease and those having the misfortune to suffer this problem are no more neurotic than most of the rest of us.

The problem has certain characteristics which will help the sufferer to make his or her own diagnosis. Usually there is a sleep disturbance starting before or coinciding with the onset of pain. There may be difficulty in getting off to sleep. The sleep may be lighter, more easily disturbed. There may be waking during the night or early morning, with difficulty in getting back to sleep. There is more tossing and turning during the night: the bedclothes are a crumpled mess in the morning. The sufferer wakes up tired, feeling he or she has not had a good night's sleep. During the day there is a loss of vitality. Daily tasks become a burden: the sufferer keeps on but this involves more effort than usual.

Such a picture could be described as that of a mild depression. The pain also has characteristics which are different to that experienced when tissue has been injured and is healing or is inflamed. It may or may not be present first thing but it characteristically gets worse later in the day. It tends to improve with exercise and is at its worst when sitting doing nothing. Sometimes vigorous exercise makes it better, at least for a time.

We are all endowed with a coping system which enables us to handle the usual environmental stresses imposed on us. We react to these stresses, whatever they may be, by doing something about them, if we can. If we cannot we adapt. This ability to adapt or cope varies considerably from individual to individual. How much this coping ability depends on our early environment and upbringing and how much it is innate (we were born that way), is not known, but by the time we have grown up it is unlikely it can be altered.

This coping system can and does get overloaded. To unload it will therefore require changes in the environment rather than in the unchangeable individual. In other words, this is not a medical problem but one of the society in which the individual lives.

In susceptible individuals this overload manifests itself in various ways. For example, it may cause what is known as the irritable bowel syndrome, nervous dyspepsia, palpitations, and so on.

When we are stressed or threatened our alerting system comes into action. We lose the ability to relax. Our sleep becomes lighter. We lose out on our deep restorative Phase 4 sleep, so we do not recharge our batteries properly, and feel tired the next day.

Another key part of this alerting system is the fusimotor nerves driving our muscle spindles. Our back and neck muscles are more prone to such increased activity. Hence the many hot painful trigger points which will not respond to any local treatment.

This problem is more common than is generally realized, and varying degrees of overload are often responsible for a neck or back pain keeping on when it should have got better. It is three times more common in women than men. This does not mean women have more vulnerable coping systems than men – probably the opposite is true. What it means is the average woman is under a bigger stress load in today's society than the average man.

It often affects the young woman who has just left school, left home, is living in a flat (often with boyfriend) and working in an office all day. It can also affect the young mother coping with youngsters on her own all day, or the solo mother, or the mother trying to hold down a demanding job as well as run a home and family, and so on. As a general rule most overloading situations happen within families, between partners, involve stresses at work, or have a financial basis.

One group of people very vulnerable to this syndrome are those who live life in what could be termed 'chronic overdrive'. You may recognize this pattern in yourself or in someone around you. These individuals are always on the go, with a mind racing two jobs ahead of the one being done. They are unable to sit still for any length of time doing nothing – the knitting needles go click click. By evening they run out of steam and like to go to bed early. They need a lot of sleep, at least eight or nine hours. Late nights play havoc with the next day. Sleep may be light and easily disturbed by the slightest sound. This pattern happens in those with a naturally very active alerting system: they need extra sleep to recharge the batteries properly. It needs little extra stress to put such an individual into the overload situation.

When a group of animals (most research has been done with rats) are crowded together into a living space smaller than they are used to in their natural surroundings they become over-stressed. There are two extremes of response to this overstress: some become withdrawn and curl up in a corner; at the other extreme some become increasingly aggressive, attacking those around them. Our response to overstress follows the same basic pattern: at the one extreme you have the withdrawn depressed individual; and at the other the aggressive angry individual who is likely to win a medal in any war.

Most of us, when overstressed, respond somewhere between these two extremes, but from experience it is the angry responders who have the greatest difficulty in overcoming this problem. To suggest they are uptight and angry does not go down too well.

Once the cause of the ongoing pain is understood by the sufferer half the battle is won. The cause or causes of the overstress have to be worked out. If anything can be done to overcome it or them it should be done. Often this is not possible: it can be difficult to get rid of one's boss, husband, or wife. One sufferer remarked that her neck pain and headaches disappeared when her husband was away on business trips. Now, what do you say to that?

The natural response to incoming stress is action. This releases the tension. Therefore more activity is needed. Whilst the trigger points in the muscles are hot this may be difficult; any activity in these muscles easily provokes more painful spasm. So to start with the activity has to be gentle and only very gradually increased; walking and swimming are often the best starters. Some initial local treatment to the trigger points may be necessary to get things going. The assistance of a physiotherapist may be needed.

Gradually, an increasingly vigorous exercise programme needs to be built up. Jogging may involve too much jarring of the spinal joints in the early stages. A rebound exerciser may be very useful so long as it is used properly. Cycling is also good, as long as there is not too much bending over low handlebars. Once it is realized that an active vigorous pain-free existence is possible, the battle has been won. It is important that a continuing programme of vigorous exercise is maintained. It is the best natural counter to stress of any sort.

Treatment

Starting from the bottom of the spine and working up:

Acute low back pain

You are struck down by a pain in or across the low back. This may be a sudden severe onset related to a known strain, or it may come on gradually after such a strain. You may feel as though something has suddenly 'gone out' in your back. Do not worry, this does not happen. This sensation is due to the sudden prising apart of the two surfaces of a facet joint.

Self help

The first thing to do is lie down, the sooner the better. In the acute stage there is a lot of painful spasm in the back muscles. These muscles are continually on the go when we are moving about and even when we are sitting. The only hope of relaxing them is to lie down. Also, lying down lowers the pressure inside the disc.

Try and find a comfortable position and stay there. Often the slightest movement hurts. As with love-making porcupines, every move has to be made with care.

The most comfortable position may be lying half face down with the upper thigh drawn well up towards the chest. Lying on one's back with the legs resting on a box, covered with cushions, is often comfortable (see Fig. 38). You may find that another position is more comfortable; do whatever is best for you.

Immediate rest is important. How long this rest should last

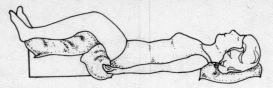

Figure 38 *How to rest with a very sore back*

depends on the severity of the attack. Except when it is thought you may have ruptured the disc, it should not be more than about three days. Remember, whilst you are resting your poor chondrocytes are not getting a square meal.

Try not to panic. Easier said than done. Take comfort from the fact that the majority of attacks get better whatever is done or not done to your back, though it may take time.

The bed

Traditional advice has been to lie on a firm mattress, if necessary putting flat boards under the mattress. The source of such advice is not known (some sadistic orthopaedic surgeon is suspected), and the rationale of such advice is hard to work out. Some say it helps. Others find it a form of torture. Some persist in spite of this: bad-tasting medicine can be more effective. By all means try boards under the mattress, but if this is more uncomfortable throw them away. Resting on a mattress on the floor may be tried, though getting up from the floor to go to the toilet is not as easy as getting out of bed. Some people's backs are more comfortable on a hard bed and some on a soft bed. If you normally find your bed comfortable and you wake up feeling rested, without back discomfort, there is no point in making a change.

At the moment water beds are the in thing. These are fine as long as there is no fear of drowning. They suit some spines but not others, so if you try one, do it on approval. It is said love-making takes on a new dimension of pleasure.

Useful tips

When we lie on our side the low back spine caves in towards the bed. This may stretch injured tissue on the underside – which will hurt. It may also compress injured tissue on the upper side – which will also hurt. This may be overcome by rolling up a bath towel and pinning it round your middle.

At least in the first twenty-four hours local cold may be more comforting than heat. Try a packet of frozen peas or crushed ice in a plastic bag, wrapped in some thin towelling. Leave it against the sore part of the back for about twenty minutes at a time. If this does not help try the opposite: local heat, in the usual form of a hot water bottle.

Traction

Self-applied traction may give a lot of relief. If there is a handy beam or bar within easy reach of the upstretched hands use it. If not, use the outer upper edge of an open door. To make it easier on your hands it helps if a rolled towel or newspaper is placed on the top of the door. With the hands firmly locked over the beam or door the trick is to lift the feet gently off the floor with the arms fully upstretched. No attempt should be made to pull oneself up with the arms. There is a muscle which goes from the shoulder down to the low back. Pulling up with the arms will cause it to tighten and thus put strain on the low back.

With the feet just off the floor all that is necessary is to hang on with the fingers and hands as long as possible, letting the rest of the body go slack. Taking the weight back on to the feet should be done as gradually as possible. A sudden jolt may provoke painful muscle spasm.

If you have gravity boots, hanging upside down may also help to relax the painful back muscles. It will certainly provide a new aspect in life, making conversation possible with the nearest sloth. It is not advised for those with heart or blood pressure problems.

Claims have been made that traction works by pulling the

joints apart and thus helping to reduce a bulging or ruptured disc. This may be so but any such beneficial effects would be very short-lasting. It is more likely the stretching of the joints and muscles stimulates sensing nerves which reflexly relax the tight painful muscles.

There is another way of applying traction which needs the help of someone else. Lie on your back with your knees and hips well flexed. Ask someone to sit side-saddle on your feet (see Fig. 39). Their fingers are then locked behind and just below your knees. If this person then leans sideways, away from you, it is possible to apply a strong pull to the back of the legs. This will pull your lower spine apart. The traction should be held for two or three minutes and then *gradually* released. Not suddenly; as this could provoke painful spasm. This may be repeated for as long as your helper can sustain the effort.

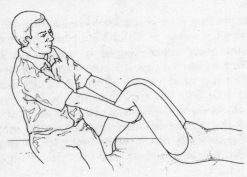

Figure 39 *How to apply steady traction to the low back:* The amount of pull should be gradually increased, then held for at least two or three minutes, and then gradually decreased.

Exercises

If the period of complete rest is only for two or three days there is no need to worry about exercises. Anyway, most exercises at this stage will be too painful. The stomach muscles very quickly lose their tone whilst in bed. Gentle frequent tightening of these is a good idea.

The back muscles are always tight and irritable. They may be gently stretched, but if this aggravates the pain it must be stopped. The following hold-relax exercise may be very useful. Lie on your back with your knees and hips bent (see Fig. 40). The head should be supported by a couple of pillows. Lock your hands at the back of the thighs, just below the knees. Gently pull your thighs back towards your chin. When this starts to feel uncomfortable, stop. Next, push against your hands with your thighs, gradually increasing the pressure. Hold on with your hands so that the thighs are prevented from straightening out. Maintain this pressure for about seven seconds (a slow count of seven), then relax. Immediately pull the thighs a little nearer to the chin, then hold still and again apply pressure. Repeat this procedure three times. The intervals between applying pressure should be as short as possible, only about three seconds.

If any muscle being contracted contains a 'hot' trigger point, or if an injured part is moved, more pain and reflex muscle spasm will result and no benefit will accrue. So, if it hurts, stop.

This hold-relax technique may not be better than applying a slow steady stretch to the muscle but it certainly takes less time. Here is how it works.

Making a muscle contract against a resistance when it is already stretched to near its limit causes maximum stimulation to the sensing nerves which measure tension – mainly the golgi tendon nerves. These have an inhibitory or dampening effect on the muscle motor nerves. This quietens down the fusimotor

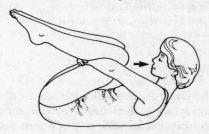

Figure 40 *Low back muscle stretch:* The knees are pulled towards the chin, not straight on to the chest.

nerves supplying the muscle spindles. As a consequence the spindles become less sensitive to stretch, and the muscle may be stretched a little further without provoking a reflex contraction. This dampening effect is short-lasting, hence the need for only a short gap between each contraction, and the need to take up the gained slack between contractions.

Once the acute stage of back pain has passed further exercises may be of help. These will be described further on.

Drugs

If the pain is acute, painkillers may give relief. Aspirin, in one form or another, is to be found in most homes. It is still one of the best mild painkillers. Aspirin may upset the stomach and cause it to bleed. It would not be a positive gain to have less pain but also a bleeding stomach ulcer, so they should be taken after food, with a drink of milk. Up to three tablets every four hours may be taken. If you experience a ringing sensation in your head your body is telling you you have had enough. If there is felt to be a need for stronger painkillers a prescription from your doctor will be necessary.

Besides straight painkillers there are three further groups of drugs which may be offered, all of doubtful value.

One is *muscle relaxants*. Any muscle relaxer strong enough to have much effect on local painful muscle spasm would likely make it difficult even to lift your little finger.

Another group is *anti-inflammation drugs*. After the average back strain if inflammation is present this is the result of tissue injury and it reflects the body's normal healing process. Dampening down such a normal reaction to injury would not necessarily be a good idea. Some pain relief may be gained at the expense of a delayed healing process. What is gained on the swings may be lost on the roundabouts. These drugs also occasionally have nasty side effects, so make sure you know what you are getting. No treatment may be the better treatment.

Another group is the *tranquillizer-antidepressant drugs*. Suffering an attack of acute back pain may cause panic — it certainly is depressing. Some tranquillizers may make the depression worse. Some antidepressants may make the muscles more tight. A large dose of a combined tranquillizer-antidepressant such as amitriptylline may help to pass the first day or two in a state of doped bliss. A significant number of attacks of back and neck pain happen at times when we are uptight and under an excessive stress load. A small dose of amitriptylline, just 10 mgms at night, may help to quieten down the overactive alerting system, and may be useful for a month or more.

Whatever you may be offered, make sure you understand what the desired effect is and what possible side effects there may be. Sleeping drugs containing any barbiturates should be avoided – barbiturates enhance the feeling of pain. Alcohol should also be avoided. A small to moderate amount also enhances pain, and you would need such a lot to dampen the pain effectively that the following morning would be pretty unpleasant.

When help is needed

There is only one emergency which may arise in an attack of low back pain, and this is very rare. If there is a massive rupture of the back wall of the disc with an extrusion of a big lump of disc material, it may trap the nerve roots inside the spinal canal, and some nerve fibres may be trapped above the level of their nerve cells. This may happen to the automatic (autonomic) nerves going to organs in the pelvis. Such entrapment may lead to death of the nerve cells, so that regeneration of the nerve fibres cannot take place. This situation requires urgent surgery to remove the lump of disc before permanent damage to the nerve cell has happened.

I must repeat: this is a very rare happening.

The main symptoms to look out for are: severe pain down both legs and a feeling of weakness in one or both legs: a numb feeling in the area which would be covered by sitting on a saddle; a loss of control of the waterworks.

Apart from this single rare emergency no further help is mandatory in most attacks of back pain. They will get better whatever you do or don't do. Many alternative treatments with offered cures are available in the open market. We will consider each of them.

A certificate for time off work will be needed by most. The boss will not appreciate a self-written sickness or accident certificate, certainly after the first week. So you have to see your own doctor.

General practitioners

During their student years doctors receive very little training on how to look after sore necks and backs and yet such problems will occupy at least ten per cent of their time when they become general practitioners. To gain expertise in all aspects of medical and surgical treatment during the years of training is impossible. Such expertise has to be acquired in post-graduate training. What little training there is in neck and back problems comes mainly from orthopaedic surgeons. These are skilled in dealing with the more serious surgical aspects of back pain, which includes less than five per cent of attacks, so the training tends to be biased.

Doctors recently qualified therefore have very little to offer to the back pain sufferer except bed rest, painkillers, or referral elsewhere.

When first starting up in general practice most doctors are soon made aware of the inadequacy of their training. I well remember, many years ago, being told in no uncertain terms that doctors in general and myself in particular were no good with backs, but a visit to so-and-so down the road soon got it fixed.

This awareness of our shortcomings has recently led to an increasing interest by the medical profession in the two main alternative treatments for neck and back problems: manipulation and acupuncture. Now an increasing number of practitioners have gained expertise in both of these modes of treatment. If your doctor is one of them you need go no further.

Manipulation

Manipulation as a form of treatment for neck and back problems has already been touched on. It has been used in the treatment of the spine and other joints for a very long time. Hippocrates, the father of medicine, described simple manipulative techniques. Crude forms of manipulation are described as part of the folk-medicine in most, if not all, cultures. In earlier times such treatment was practised by the original orthopaedic surgeons, the bone setters; the skills were often handed down from father to son.

With the advent of modern scientific medicine in the middle of last century, manipulative treatment was discarded by the orthodox medical profession. At this time tuberculosis was rampant. This often led to abscesses in bones and joints. Horrific stories of what had happened to such bones and joints after manipulation were enough to deter most doctors, and doctors who still practised manipulation were regarded as beyond the pale.

This form of treatment was soon taken over by others outside the medical profession. First came the osteopaths and then the chiropractors, both starting in America. They both built up their own training schools. The American osteopaths have gradually upgraded their standards of training so that now the degree of DO (Doctor of Osteopathy) is on a par with MD (Doctor of Medicine) in most American states. As well as having similar medical training to MDs, DOs are also trained in the skills of manipulation. Now, a lot of qualified DOs practise little if any manipulative treatment. They have followed specialized training courses and have become surgeons, gynaecologists, specialist physicians, and so on, as happens with MDs. From personal experience, the American-trained osteopaths still practising manipulation are very good indeed: probably the best in the world. Their evangelical zeal has been tempered by the fire (or should it be the cold water?) of orthodox scientific medicine.

It is still possible to call yourself an osteopath without specific qualifications, and you would be well advised to take great care in the selection of your manipulator.

*

If one's house has a lot of glass on the outside second thoughts are necessary if one has the urge to throw a stone. This is the case when discussing chiropractic.

Both the osteopathic and chiropractic professions started out as anti-orthodox-medicine movements. At that time there was some widespread dissaffection with what was offered, or not able to be offered, by doctors. A pole tends to create a counterpole. In order to sell this counterpole exaggerated claims were made for what manipulation could cure. The reason for this was largely the responsibility of the medical profession and due to diagnostic mistakes made by doctors.

A patient would complain of a pain in the region of the gall bladder, on the right side of the front of the stomach, just below the ribs. He or she would be told by the doctor that the gall bladder was diseased. A visit to the chiropractor and a few manipulations of the dorsal spine would result in the disappearence of the pain. Thus, the chiropractor had cured 'gall bladder disease' and rightly claimed that he could do so in others. Fortunately, such errors in diagnosis are now less common. Referred pain is better understood and modern tests are better able to tell what is diseased and what is not.

In order to sell a product alternative to orthodox medicine, it was necessary to learn the tricks of the hard sell. An important part of chiropractic training is the teaching of communication and the art of selling what one has to offer.

When we are sick and/or in pain we tend to be frightened, fearful of the unknown, and desperately want to get better. If we see someone who tells us they know exactly what the problem is, such and such a vertebra is out of place, and that they can fix it by doing so and so, a lot of confidence is generated. At the very least this provokes a very good enhanced placebo response.

If, on the other hand, we see someone who tells us they cannot be sure what exactly is wrong with us but that this form of treatment may help and if it does not something else will be tried, not much confidence is generated and treatment is less likely to be effective.

*

Perhaps this is one of the directions in which modern medicine has gone a little off the rails.

When dealing with most back and neck problems we are coping with an ageing process, not a disease, which has become painful for one reason or another. One of the reasons it started and continues to hurt is because we are uptight. If we did not start out uptight we certainly become so because of the ongoing pain. This helps to initiate and perpetuate the pain—muscle spasm—pain cycle. If we consult someone who seems to understand our problem and offers a sure fire cure this uptightness is diminished and the body's natural placebo response is likely to be stimulated. The vicious circle may then be broken.

This enhanced placebo response is a very powerful weapon in helping those in pain. If there is no cure for the cause of pain its use should be invoked wherever possible. The doctor should step off his/her pedestal and make closer contact with patients. There is a need for the return to Desmond Morris's 'tribal backscratcher' role.

It is not the intent to pass judgement on the chiropractic profession. There is no doubt they have been able to relieve many patients who were not helped by orthodox medicine. The reverse is also true. They have filled a gap in the caring business which has been largely ignored by doctors, though this is changing as their undergraduate training has slowly improved.

With increasing knowledge chiropractors' exaggerated claims are diminishing. Their anti-doctor stance is lessening, just as doctors have become less suspicious of them. Gradually communication between the two professions is improving: '*Fas est hoste doceri*' (it is right to be taught by the enemy). Probably they will eventually suffer the same fate as the American osteopaths, though an anti-doctor stance has good marketing value.

Chiropractors are well trained in the art of manipulation before they graduate, whereas doctors and physiotherapists have to learn these skills after graduation. Because they had little else to offer in the past there has been a tendency to overuse manipulation. There is now good evidence that it either works quickly or not at all. So, if you visit a chiropractor and you feel there has been no improvement after, at the most, three treatments it is then time to make a rapid exit.

Nowadays, manipulative treatment may be available from some doctors. If not, the doctor may refer you to a physiotherapist. All qualified physiotherapists have had no basic pre-registration training in manipulation, but there are comprehensive post-registration courses on the subject for those who wish to specialize, and most physiotherapists out in practice are adequately trained in manipulation.

You may decide to go to a chiropractor instead. If you do it is a good general principle to keep the knowledge of such visits from your doctor. Such information may threaten your doctor's health, causing a marked rise in blood pressure.

What is manipulation?   Manipulation is a word which conjures up different meanings to different people. According to my dictionary, manipulation is the shrewd or devious effort to manage or influence for one's own purpose. In other words, one of life's games. Besides this general definition, medical manipulation is defined as the therapeutic movement of bones and other tissues by the use of the hands. The elbows, knees, chest, and maybe feet, could also be included.

There are several different schools of manipulation, teaching different techniques. These vary from the rather violent to the very gentle. The advocates of these varying techniques share a common enthusiasm for their own methods.

Some techniques are described as osteopathic or chiropractic. In fact, most techniques have been pinched from somewhere else, and a lot have been handed down for generations.

One of the common techniques employed by most of the different schools is joint 'popping' manipulation. As the sufferer is being manipulated a 'click' or 'clicks' can be heard coming from the spine. This is very suggestive of something going back into place: 'My back was out. Now it is back in place.' Nothing could be further from the truth.

If a finger is pulled on with sufficient force, a similar 'click' may be heard. Some people can do this more easily than others. It is known as 'knuckle cracking', and this is what happens. The sudden forceful separation of the two joint surfaces creates an increased negative pressure inside the joint. The joint surfaces are separated from each other by a thin film of fluid, the synovial fluid. When this negative pressure reaches a certain level the fluid is vapourized. Tiny bubbles of gas are produced. It is the bursting of these bubbles that creates the noise.

The trick of joint 'popping' is to place the subject in such a position that a force may be applied to the facet joints as near to right angles to their surfaces as is possible. It is easier to do if the joint surfaces are in full apposition to each other, neither bent forward nor bent back. The force then applied has to be very sudden – what is called a high velocity, short amplitude thrust. If a steady force was applied the natural joint tightness and resisting muscle action would prevent the cavitation effect. This cavitation effect, producing the 'click', involves very little movement of the joint: only a doubling of the joint space. To perform this type of manipulation requires quick reflexes in the manipulator. He or she has to apply the sudden high-velocity thrust before any reflex protective muscle action takes place.

Looking again at the alignment of the facet joints in the different regions of the spine it will be seen that different movements will be required to achieve the gapping or cavitation effect. For instance, in the low back a twisting movement will be most effective (see Fig. 41).

In the middle part of the thoracic (chest) spine a direct thrust from the back directed through to the front of the chest will tend to prize apart the facet joints, pushing the surface coming from the lower vertebra away from that coming from the upper (see Fig. 42).

In the neck the thrust will need to be in a different direction. If you side bend your neck one way it will jam the facet joints together on the side to which you are bending, and tend to prise apart the facet joints on the other. If you now twist your neck round in the opposite direction you will find you cannot turn it round very far. This movement tends to further jam together the facets on one side and prise them apart on the other. All

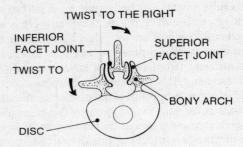

Figure 41 *Cross section of a low back facet joint:* Twisting the lower joint surface one way and the upper the other will tend to prize apart one joint and jam the other together.

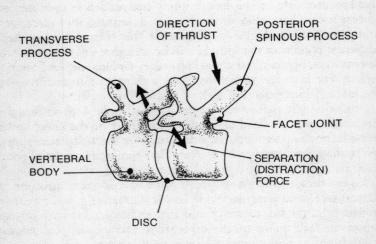

Figure 42 *Manipulation of the thoracic (chest) spine:* A direct thrust down on the vertebra below will tend to prize apart the facet joints above.

that is now required is a sudden sharp increase in the side bend and/or twist in the opposite direction and the facet joints will 'pop'.

Some techniques of manipulation involve sudden violent thrusts over the spinal joints. Others utilize traction on the joints, pulling them apart. More gentle techniques employ rhythmic movement to the joints, so-called mobilization techniques. A further group work specifically on the muscles, stretching them out by one means or another. Still others just work on the trigger points.

All these techniques have their own circle of devotees, and so must be effective in a significant proportion of instances. Therefore the question to be asked is: what can they possibly have in common? Of course, they will all tend to provoke the enhanced placebo response, but do they do anything else? The short answer to this is, Yes.

Theories abound on how manipulation works. Some of these have already been mentioned. The commonly used techniques involve an attack on the joints, so possible problems within the joints that could be relieved by joint 'popping' have been looked for, such as trapped synovial fringes, jammed joints, trapped meniscoids, trapped loose fragments of cartilage. It is unlikely any of these situations could account for more than a very few incidences of neck and back pain. A sudden increase in the negative pressure within the facet joint would in fact tend to suck anything between the two surfaces even further in.

During joint popping the amount of movement within the joint is very small – only a doubling of the normal joint space – and the two surfaces immediately spring back together again. Anyhow, other techniques not involving joint popping also seem to be equally effective or ineffective on occasions.

Certainly, from what is now known about the structure of our discs, it is more than unlikely manipulation would have any lasting effect on anything which may have gone wrong with them. And manipulation will have no beneficial effect on damaged healing tissue, probably the opposite.

What in fact manipulation of the facet joints can do, and probably only does, is reflexly to relax tight painful muscle. That it can do this has been adequately demonstrated in scientifically acceptable experiments.

In other words, by manipulating the joints the muscles are conned into relaxing. Remember, the casing of the facet joints and surrounds contains many sensing nerves, so the manipulation either stimulates sensing nerves which inhibit the muscle spindle fusimotor nerves, the large golgi tendon organs and Type 3 joint sensing nerves, or blocks input from nerves which may excite the fusimotor nerves, mainly the Type 1 joint sensing nerves.

This explains why so many different techniques may be equally effective, or at times ineffective. It also probably means that those with a high degree of manipulative skill are not necessarily more effective than those with lesser skills, as long as the right part of the spine is manipulated. In my personal experience, increasing expertise over the years did not seem to improve effectiveness to any noticeable degree, though there was improvement in knowing when, when not to, and where to manipulate.

This also means quite a high percentage of our attacks of neck and back pain do not involve appreciable tissue damage. Sensing nerves which excite muscle may be stimulated, which initiates the painful muscle spasm. This then becomes a self-perpetuating vicious circle, perpetuated further by general overall uptightness and also possible increased sensing input from locally worn joints.

So by all means have your neck or back manipulated and/or your trigger points treated by whomever you choose. But remember, such treatment will work quickly or not at all. The question now is when you should have such treatment. As a general rule, if you can get to whomever you are going to see without too much discomfort, it is OK to go ahead.

When not to have manipulation The time not to be manipulated is when any tissue injury has taken place, for instance a disc rupture or a ligament tear. There is no way in which the moving of injured tissue could be helpful; more probably it will do further damage. Injured tissue has to pass through the normal healing process, and until it is healed will be a potential source of discomfort.

So, you must try and distinguish between pain caused by tissue injury and that coming from painful muscle spasm. Unfortunately, there is no clear-cut distinction between the two — it is just a matter of degree. Inflammation (reaction to tissue injury) pain tends to be more severe and keeps on keeping on until the healing process is complete, while the other shows much more fluctuation. Stimulation of the pain-sensing nerves by a reaction to injury will also cause reflex spasm in related muscles which may be a source of further pain. If the sufferer is tense or upset, this may complicate the situation by helping to perpetuate the muscle spasm, and thus make a successful outcome to manipulation less likely.

Taking these factors into account, manipulation is less likely to help in the following situations:

1   If the pain does not ease within a few minutes of resting, and if strong painkillers are needed to get any sleep.

2   If the pain wakes you in the night, particularly after only an hour or two of sleep, and if it is then difficult getting back to sleep, because of pain. If you have to get up and move about for some time before sleep is again possible, then manipulation is definitely out.

   A sudden movement whilst sleeping may provoke painful muscle spasm, causing waking. This quickly abates and it is soon possible to get back to sleep. This is not an indication against manipulation.

   If there is waking during the night and difficulty getting back to sleep, but not because of pain, the problem is one of an overactive alerting system which may not respond to manipulation.

3   An inflammation (reaction to injury) pain is always particularly bad first thing in the morning, when you are trying to get out of bed. This constant nagging soreness has to be distinguished from that caused by painful stiff muscles. If the pain is from stiff muscles it is possible to move without too much discomfort as long as great care is taken. This painful stiffness quickly eases off with movement, say in half

an hour. If the pain takes an hour or more to ease off, and then does not ease off to any appreciable extent, manipulation is very unlikely to help. Inflammation and possibly uptightness is responsible.

4   If there is virtual freedom from pain after a night's sleep and the pain comes on during the day, depending on what you do, manipulation will not solve the problem. Immediate relief may occur, because tight painful muscles have been reflexly relaxed, but this will be short-lasting. This short-lasting relief is a trap for the unwary and is responsible for a lot of futile manipulation. The stresses of the day, both physical and emotional, are responsible for the provocation of pain. These have to be attended to before any lasting relief will occur.

5   If all activities – walking, standing, sitting, bending – during the day are painful if persisted in for more than a short time, and if lying down only gives relief after some time, inflammation should be suspected and manipulation should be avoided.

6   If the pain spreads in a continuous line down the thigh and leg, even into the foot, within a matter of a few hours or a day or so, a disc rupture should be suspected and manipulation will not help.

Sometimes, if the lump of broken-off disc material remains at the centre of the back of the disc, the resulting pain may remain just in the back. In this situation manipulation, using a technique involving a twist, may move this lump of loose disc outwards so that it may irritate the nerve roots going out the side of the spine. This may cause the severe back pain to disappear and instead become a severe thigh and leg pain. Such a situation has been known to occur and there is no need for undue concern. At least, the diagnosis has been clarified and immediate relief may now be obtained from surgery. It will also cause delight to some orthopaedic surgeons who will point out what a dreadful business manipulation is. Such folk must have very little glass in their house, with no attached greenhouse.

Often it may be difficult to decide if there has been any tissue injury, particularly if this is very minor. In this situation manipulation has to be tried – no guarantees offered. If it works, well and good. If not, nothing has been lost but it should be quickly abandoned.

If you are fully conscious and able to tell the manipulator which movement hurts and which does not, no lasting harm can result and useful information will be gained.

Immediately after a successful manipulation there should be some pain relief and an ability to move further. For instance, it may now be possible to touch your toes. Discomfort may again flare up later the same day. This is often a different discomfort to the original, and gradually settles over the next two days. If manipulation is going to be successful a maximum of three to four treatments are all that should be necessary.

Dangers of manipulation   In the low back there is only one very slight possible risk attached to manipulation. In the presence of a disc rupture a forceful movement to the low back may squeeze out more disc material which may threaten the nerve roots travelling down inside the spinal canal. Such a possibility has already been described, and it calls for immediate surgery, to remove the offending lump of disc.

It is a very, very rare happening. In my own experience of nearly twenty years of looking after many thousands of low back problems it has only happened in three patients. In two of these it happened spontaneously, no hand had been laid upon them, and in the other it happened during a manipulation whilst the patient was anaesthetized (I might add, by someone else). All were completely relieved by immediate surgery.

In the neck there is one potentially life-threatening risk in having manipulation: the risk of damaging one of the two arteries which travel up the neck in a bony canal on each side of the spine. As we saw earlier (page 71), these arteries hook over the sides of the first vertebra (the atlas) before entering the hole in the base of the skull. They supply blood to part of the brain.

Very occasionally some people are born with one of these

arteries much smaller than the other. They may be at risk from manipulation, if the larger of the two arteries suffers damage. This damage may occur if the neck is subjected to a violent twist whilst held in the extended (bent back) position. It has also happened spontaneously, when someone has suddenly looked back over the shoulder whilst backing a car.

There is a simple test which will determine most of those at risk. This should be done by all those who manipulate necks. Make sure if anyone offers to manipulate your neck they first do the following:

While lying on your back on a couch, your head should be allowed to bend backwards to its full extent over the end of the couch. Your neck should then be gently turned one way to its full extent and held there for a few seconds, and then turned fully in the opposite direction and again held there for a few seconds. If these positions make you feel very giddy, sick, faint, or cause double vision, it will be wise to call it a day.

As a general rule there should be no risk if no manipulations are done with the neck held backwards and then twisted. Taking into account the millions of neck manipulations taking place every day, the risks of this damage are very small. Nevertheless, the risk is there – there are scattered reports of such happenings in different medical journals, invariably caused by some poor chiropractor. If equivalent notice was taken of daily medical and surgical misadventures, a few extra medical journals would be needed.

We get back to the glasshouse stone-throwing business.

In justification it should be pointed out that it is only the rare cases that are sufficiently newsworthy to persuade medical journal editors to publish the details.

There is one other danger attached to manipulation which is in no way life threatening. I understand that if you have your hair cut whilst staying in Singapore, the barber, after finishing the haircut, will deftly side bend your neck one way, twist it the other, and then with a quick flick will 'pop' your neck facet joints. You experience a whole barrage of clicks in your neck. This results in an immediate feeling of wellbeing, which will last while paying the bill and walking away down the street, but not for much longer.

Spine facet joints not in a painful area of the back are much easier to 'pop' than those that are: they are not held together to the same extent by protective muscle spasm. Nevertheless, 'popping' these symptomless joints does reflexly relax the associated muscles, and our neck and shoulder girdle muscles are notorious for getting uptight to a lesser or greater extent. These reflexly relaxed muscles are directly responsible for the feeling of well being which is one of the reasons for the long-standing popularity of manipulation: we feel better afterwards, at least for a time. If there is associated relief from pain well and good, but if the relief does not last for long, manipulation is not serving any useful purpose, and frequently-manipulated joints seem to become increasingly unstable. You feel the need for more frequent manipulations, until eventually there is a real danger of ending up in a worse state than when you started.

If your joints 'pop' very easily, it is likely that the wrong ones are being manipulated. Some people with very loose joints learn the trick of 'popping' their own. It may become a bit of an obsession, like Knuckle cracking.

To summarize Manipulation is likely to be of help for up to a month after the onset of pain: after this time it may be less effective. Trigger points tend to develop slowly. After the first two weeks a combination of manipulation and local trigger point treatment is probably best. After a month or so trigger point treatment alone is probably best, and this should be combined with stretch exercises for the muscles containing the trigger points.

Another way of helping yourself

A physiotherapist in New Zealand, Robin McKenzie, made a chance discovery. A patient of his, suffering from acute low back pain, was left accidentally on his own in one of the treatment rooms lying on his stomach with his back slightly arched. Such a position was regarded as very bad for someone with back pain. When his presence was remembered a mad rush back was made, expecting to find him in great discomfort. In fact, he was a lot better. Since then, working on a trial and error basis, McKenzie has found about seventy per cent of his patients with acute low back pain could be helped by a programme of gradual passive, not active, back extension (bending backwards).

This is a very simple non-traumatic way to deal with your back pain, fully described in McKenzie's book *Treat Your Own Back*, and there is no reason why you should not give it a go. Here is what you do:

Lie on your stomach without a pillow. To start with this may be too uncomfortable, since it causes the low back to arch backwards, so place two or three thin cushions under your stomach, enough to allow the low back to bend forward into a comfortable position. Stay in this position for ten minutes. Then remove, or get someone to remove, one of the pillows. Then stay in the new position for a further ten minutes. Then remove a further pillow, and so on. When you have been lying flat for about ten minutes, gradually push yourself up with your arms and place a pillow under the top of your chest. This will gradually increase the backward arch in your low back. Then rest for ten minutes. One or two more pillows may be gradually added until your back is fully arched backwards. After ten minutes with the back fully arched and if it feels quite comfortable it is time to get up. When doing so it is important to maintain the backward arching at all times. Every waking hour for the next two or three days you should place your hands on your hips and arch backwards as far as possible, holding this position for about three minutes.

When the initial pain is severe it may travel down the back of one thigh, and be associated with a side bend and twist of the low spine, the side bend usually being away from the painful side. Anyone standing behind you can observe the bend and twist. This situation is called a sciatic scoliosis (sciatic = leg pain, scoliosis = side bend).

It was thought this painful side bend was due to a lump of ruptured disc which was pressing on the side of a nerve root, and the reflex side bend was an attempt to get away from this irritation. This is unlikely: it would not explain why such a side bend often immediately disappears when the sufferer lies down, nor the fact that rapid relief is often achieved. There is no way in which rapid relief could be possible in the presence of a recently extruded lump of disc associated with an inflammatory reaction to injury.

Such a deformity can be explained by irritable spasm in one particular muscle, called the iliopsoas muscle (see Fig. 43). The iliopsoas muscles, one on each side, arise from the sides of the front of the low back spine and also the inside of the back of the pelvis, and are inserted into the inside of the top of the thigh bone (femur). A pull on the muscle's origin from the spine will tend to increase the sway in the low back, whilst a pull on its insertion into the thigh will tend to pull the thigh forwards and also turn it outwards. If, when standing, one of these muscles is pulling more than the other it will cause the low back to be pulled forward more on one side. This will cause a side bend

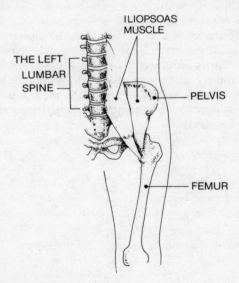

Figure 43 *The Iliopsoas muscle*

and twist. If both are painfully tight it will make arching backwards very painful.

From experience, stretching out this muscle seems to be as effective as doing the slow passive backward bending. Also, if a hold-relax technique is used it is much quicker.

This is what you do.

Carefully get down on your hands and knees (see Fig. 44). If one side is more painful than the other, gently slide the knee on the painful side backwards and the other knee forwards. As the thigh on the painful side is slowly straightened it will put the iliopsoas muscle on that side on the stretch. When the limit of comfortable stretch is reached, push down with this backward knee, using a steady pressure. Hold this pressure for a slow count of seven, then relax. Immediately slide the knee further back and the other one further forward and then repeat the steady downward pressure for a further seven seconds. The time gap between applying each pressure should be as short as possible, not more than three seconds. When the knees will go no further back or forward it is possible to increase the stretch on the muscle by arching the head and shoulders further back. The amount of increased stretch applied to the muscle each time should be small. If you stretch too much, painful spasm may be provoked. If it hurts, immediately reduce the stretch, or give it up for a time and try again later. Both sides should be stretched. As with the McKenzie technique, once the muscle is stretched out this stretch needs to be maintained, and frequent arching backwards is necessary.

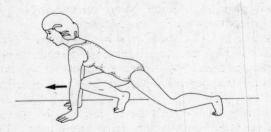

Figure 44 *The Iliopsoas muscle stretch*

It has been suggested that back pain is caused by increased internal pressure on the back wall of the disc, and that the slow extension relieves this pressure by pushing the contents of the disc forwards. If this is so, why does it need to be done so slowly? The slow bending backwards technique is claimed to work in about seventy per cent of attacks of low back pain. This, coupled with the claims of those using quite different techniques, including acupuncture, would in fact strongly suggest that in approximately seventy per cent of attacks of back pain the main culprit is painful muscle spasm. This is probably provoked by very minor strains of the back joints which are not sufficient to provoke a significant reaction to injury (inflammation).

Acupuncture

Over the past few years acupuncture as a treatment for all sorts of problems has really taken off. In the early 1970s, when China opened her doors to Western journalists and statesmen, they were seen to be using acupuncture to anaesthetize patients for surgical operations. One American journalist had his appendix removed while acupuncture rather than general anaesthesia was used. Since then doctors and others have flocked to China to learn all about acupuncture, while Chinese doctors have flocked to the West to learn all about modern anaesthesia.

In China acupuncture has been a standard treatment for generations. There was little else to offer. The Chinese have evolved highly complex acupuncture point charts, with different points assigned to different body functions. These bear no relation to any known nerve connections.

Modifications of acupuncture have evolved. Now, some acupuncturists pass electric currents through the inserted needles (electro-acupuncture). Others have found that the insertion of needles into the outer coating of bones is effective (osteo-acupuncture).

Acupuncture has recently been, and still is, the subject of intensive scientific investigation. There seems little doubt the act of inserting needles into someone is capable of provoking the release of the body's own natural painkillers, the so-called endorphins, which also impart a sense of well being. Then again, so does a brisk run around the block.

Clinical trials of its effectiveness have been carried out. So far, the results do not show a benefit significantly better than that expected from the enhanced placebo response: sixty to seventy per cent improvement.

Then again, if you can offer someone who is suffering from a pain not caused by any disease, as is the case in most neck and back pain, a sixty to seventy per cent chance of relief by sticking pins in them at specific sites, the odds are far better than doing nothing at all.

As already mentioned, the significant co-relationship between the sites of traditional Chinese acupuncture points and the known sites of trigger points is of interest. Obviously the Chinese doctors have by chance found these sites to be effective in giving relief. A needle inserted into a trigger point provokes local muscle contraction and a definite unpleasant sensation. This may reflexly stimulate the production of the body's endorphins or it may be suggestive to the sufferer that something potentially beneficial is going on, thus provoking the enhanced placebo response, which will have the same effect.

Ritual behaviour has been known to be of instinctive value and benefit to humankind for a very long time. Religion, the State and medicine have taken advantage of this fact. It would seem any ritual, the more complex the better, is a potent stimulator of the enhanced placebo response, and taking part in any ritual has the potential to make us feel good. Probably a large part of the beneficial effect of acupuncture is dependent on the associated ritual. There is no harm in that. It is an unfortunate paradox that as acupuncture becomes increasingly demystified it will probably become less effective.

The main danger of acupuncture is that the sufferer is a passive receiver of benefit – if the pain goes he or she is cured. This is not so. There is no disease to cure. Any active steps necessary to prevent a recurrence will tend to be ignored. The discipline required to help oneself further will be forgotten.

Acupuncture is claimed to be very effective immediately after the onset of back pain. It is understood Chinese factories have a resident acupuncturist: you hurt your back at work – straight to the acupuncturist – straight back to work.

That it may be effective again highlights the fact that the majority of attacks of acute low back pain are due to sudden painful muscle spasm. Acupuncture, like manipulation and any other treatment, would certainly not cause the disappearance of injured tissue.

So, if you wish to give acupuncture a go, the sooner the better. An increasing number of doctors have become aware of their inadequacies when dealing with pain syndromes which have no known underlying disease. Many have become skilled in manipulation, acupuncture, and so on. If possible, you should turn to one of these doctors rather than to any self-styled expert acupuncturist. The skilled insertion of needles may be no better, but the ability to diagnose the problem and to spot any possible ominous disease will be.

Treatment of a disc rupture

So, you are struck down with severe back pain which soon spreads down one leg, and a ruptured disc is suspected.

You have two choices: either sit it out, or more correctly, lie it out, or have the offending piece of disc removed. Prolonged bed rest has its own particular hazard – remember your poor starving chondrocytes. Some mobilization as soon as possible would be wise; gentle walking about as soon as possible. If you can get hold of one, a lumbar corset may help. Corsets do not effectively immobilize the low back but they do give some support.

If surgery is contemplated it will be necessary to see an orthopaedic surgeon. Orthopaedic surgeons vary in their enthusiasm for back surgery, and their techniques also vary. As a general rule the longer they have lived with those they have operated on the more reluctant they become to operate. The reasons for this are obvious: no surgery can alter the already present joint wear and tear. The piece of disc which is causing the immediate problem may be removed, but what about all the bits of disc found in post mortems on people with no significant history of back troubles? Long term follow-ups (seven to ten years), suggest that those who have had surgery are not appreciably better off in the long run than those who were treated medically. They seem just as likely to get problems in the future. It would thus seem the best surgery can offer is rapid relief from the current severe pain. This, of course, may be sufficient to justify its use.

There are two different surgical approaches to the disc:

Laminectomy   Getting to the back wall of the disc is difficult. To make it easier, a window is cut out of the bone of the back wall of the lamina, hence the name laminectomy (see Fig. 45). Once this is done the nerve roots can be moved aside and the back wall of the disc may be seen. Any lumps of disc may then be removed.

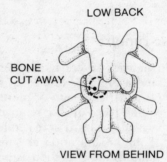

Figure 45 *Laminectomy:* The back view of the low back spine showing where the bone is cut out. This allows the surgeon to get a better view of the back of the disc.

Discectomy   This is becoming the operation of choice for many orthopaedic surgeons. No bone is removed, so there is minimum tissue disturbance. Entry to the disc is gained by cutting through the gap at the centre of the back between each vertebra, which means cutting through the ligamentum flavum. This gives only limited access. In order to see the back of the disc the nerve roots have to be pulled aside. Occasionally this has caused damage to the nerve roots, but this should not happen if the surgeon is experienced.

In summary, if I had the misfortune to rupture a disc and the question of an operation arose, I would choose a well matured orthopaedic surgeon who had spent some time on the track and who was also skilled at doing discectomies.

If there is doubt about the advisability of surgery, special X-rays may be asked for. As already explained, ordinary X-rays do not show up the outline of the discs. The spinal canal may be outlined for a special X-ray by injecting radio-opaque dyes. These are reasonably reliable in showing up bulges of the back wall of the disc, but they can be a bit unpleasant and they occasionally cause side effects. The latest CAT scan is the most reliable, completely harmless way of obtaining the necessary information, but it is expensive.

Sometimes, these X-rays are necessary to make absolutely sure there *is* a piece of disc which needs removing. Sometimes they are used because it is impossible to be sure on clinical examination alone *which* disc is responsible for the pain. If X-rays are not taken and the surgeon 'goes in blind', he or she may have to explore two discs if the first guess is wrong. This is obviously something to be avoided if possible.

Indications for surgery

The generally accepted indications for surgery are as follows:
1 A persistent severe pain in the back and down one leg which does not improve with adequate rest, associated with clear evidence of nerve root entrapment: that is, persistent marked painful restriction of straight leg raising, loss of reflex response, usually the ankle reflex, muscle weakness and wasting. It takes time for muscle wasting to become evident, and as long as the pain is getting less, it is not of undue concern. Remember, the damage has been done and cannot

be undone. Regeneration of the damaged nerve fibres will take place but it takes a long time. The lump of extruded disc material will gradually shrink as the reaction to injury subsides. This will take pressure off the nerve and thus allow regeneration.

The body's reaction to the injury, depending on the size of the lump of disc material, eventually leads either to its complete absorption and disappearance or to its conversion into a shrunken inert lump of fibrous tissue.

Depending on its size, this may take up to three months. A severe pain persisting for longer than this must mean something else is going on. This usually means ongoing painful muscle spasm which was initially provoked by the reaction to the injury and which is still persisting because of an ongoing overactive alerting system.

2 Economic considerations. When there is no way in which you can afford the necessary time off work to allow natural healing. This may be particularly so for those who have to run their own business, the self-employed: the longer the disability goes on the greater the anxiety. The greater the anxiety the more uptight we become, and the more likely is persistence of the pain.

Any further indications for surgery are not absolute. They depend on the enthusiasm of the surgeon and on the response he may make to the pressures you might impose on him.

Alternative orthopaedic treatment

Chymopapain injections   Chymopapain is an enzyme similar to that used to tenderize meat. When injected into a disc it digests the proteoglycans which have been manufactured by the chondrocytes. The chondrocytes themselves are not affected and it takes them about two years to manufacture enough new proteoglycans to replace those which were destroyed. The injection of chymopapain leads to the collapse of the bulging disc. This will take the pressure off a compromised nerve root.

Chymopapain injections are an alternative to disc surgery but are not universally accepted as such, particularly in America. The treatment can be very painful for a short time and it is unpredictable in effect, though this may be due to incorrect selection of suitable subjects. It has possible side effects, the potentially most serious being a severe life-threatening allergic reaction. As this danger is known, adequate counter-measures should be available.

Chymopapain is said to be an effective alternative to surgery in about seventy per cent of cases. It has the great advantage of not involving any surgical damage to tissue.

Epidural steroid injections   Steroids are manufactured chemicals which have a similar structure to naturally occuring body hormones. These hormones are, amongst other things, the body's natural anti-inflammation agents. If steroids are carefully injected into the spinal canal round the nerve roots which are involved in a reaction to injury, they may be very effective in reducing this reaction and thus relieve the chemically induced pain. Because the reaction is taking place in the first few weeks after injury this is the time when the injections are more likely to be effective. They should, if possible, be used in the first six weeks after the onset of pain. Of course, they will not be effective if the disc is just bulging and has not ruptured. Their effectiveness thus depends on the accuracy of the diagnosis.

Traction   If you are confined to bed in hospital, some orthopaedic surgeons still recommend continous traction. You are attached to a rope running over a pulley at the end of the bed with weights hanging down. The foot of the bed is raised in order to provide a counter-weight. The amount of weight which can be applied in such a position is not very effective in pulling your low back joints apart. By maintaining a steady pressure and by further restricting any movement such traction is effectively interfering with chondrocyte nutrition; you may have to pay the price for this later. It certainly has the effect of pinning you down in one place, making it difficult to rush off for advice elsewhere. Intermittent traction may be effective in relieving painful muscle spasm. As we have already seen, you can do this yourself.

If offered continous traction you should decline, as politely as possible.

Plaster-of-Paris jackets At one time these used to be a popular form of torture and are still occasionally offered as treatment. In order to effectively immobilize one joint in your back it is necessary to immobilize just about every other joint. You are immobilized by a complete surrounding of plaster-of-Paris from just below the armpits to your bottom. This may allow you to move about with less pain, but at a price.

Immobilizing joints, particularly spinal joints, has the drawback of shutting down the activity of most of the joint-casing sensing nerves. If this goes on for long enough the nerves not being used just fade away: a part of our integrated information feedback system will be lost. Again, we may pay a price later.

If you have the misfortune to be offered one of these plaster-of-Paris jackets I would suggest a polite refusal.

Corsets These come in various shapes and sizes. The usual ones provide a support from the buttocks to the lower rib cage, and most have metal rod stiffeners at the back, which can be moulded to a shape which is comfortable to the sufferer.

These supports may be of great value immediately after a back strain. They help to increase pressure inside the abdomen which has the effect of unloading some of the strain on the back joints. They do not totally limit movement in the joints of the low back, which is a good thing, but they do cause some restriction, which is also a good thing.

Those of us with well-rounded curves are often best suited to corsets. The bony ones may find them too uncomfortable.

As a general rule they should not be used for more than a few weeks, otherwise they may lead to further weakness of the abdominal muscles which are our natural back brace. It is wise to do abdominal muscle strengthening exercises while using a corset. There is also a danger they may become an emblem of our suffering and they have been known to be used by the wearer as a subtle tool to manipulate those nearest and dearest.

One of the great advantages of a corset, and one that I have rarely seen mentioned, is that it helps the sufferer to reprogramme his or her habitual way of bending. It is impossible to use the back joints to any great extent so more use has to be made of the hips and knees. After you have abandoned your corset you should continue to pretend to yourself it is still there whenever any bending is done.

Some people who lead strenuous physical lives may be protected by wearing their corset at the times they expect increased stress on their back.

Occasionally, people find the corset makes their back pain worse, particularly when they try to do any bending. Often, this may be because there are overstressed joints above those being supported by the corset. This is usually at the junction between the chest (thoracic) and low back (lumbar) spine. As explained before, this is often the site of increased wear and tear. Strained joints in this region may be responsible for pain in the low back. When bending, because of the relative restriction of the low back joints, the joints above the restriction tend to get used more than is usual. Thus they may hurt more if they are already under stress. Therefore, if a corset aggravates the pain the situation should be reassessed. Your back pain may in fact be coming from these higher joints. There will be local tenderness and stiffness in the joints plus very tender trigger points in the back muscles level with the joints.

This part of the spine, and the low back, can be effectively immobilized by getting someone to strap your back in the following manner:

Buy a roll of non-elastic strapping, 5 cm wide. While standing up straight, get someone to apply two strips of strapping going from the top of the shoulders and crossing over to half way down the opposite buttock (see Fig. 46). The two strips should cross at about the level of the low chest part of the spine. Such strapping is usually tolerable for about three days. If it does not lead to rapid relief it should be abandoned. If it does lead to relief it may be replaced for as long as is necessary. Some skins

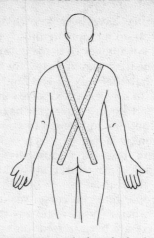

Figure 46 *Non-elastic strapping applied to the back*

are sensitive to the strapping and become very itchy, in which case it has to be abandoned.

So, we have looked at all the things you can do for yourself, and what can be done to you by others, if you have had the misfortune to suffer a disc rupture.

No active manual treatment to the joints will help while a reaction to injury is taking place. Treatment such as manipulation and local trigger point treatment may be of value later, when the reaction to injury dies down, and any ongoing pain may be due to residual painful muscle spasm. Depending on the severity of the rupture, say in four to eight weeks after the onset of pain, when sleeping at night is much better and the daytime pain is not so severe and more intermittent, then you can try manipulation.

Acute pain from the neck and thoracic (chest) spine

The overall management of acute low back pain has been described at some lenth. Long-term management and further general advice will be covered in the section on prevention and exercises (pp. 159–194).

Painful episodes coming from other regions of the spine, with one exception, tend to be less severe and incapacitating. The same general principles of management apply to them. Except in those coming from the low neck, most of the attacks are due to minor overstress of joints which already show some wear and tear. Any ongoing pain usually relates to the development of hot trigger points. The areas where pain may be experienced from these regions of the spine have already been described. The response to local treatment, either by local trigger point treatment, manipulation, or both, is usually good. There is no reason why you should not get someone to have a go at the trigger points. Where they are likely to be found has been described.

If local pressuring is used remember the following rules:

If the pressuring is exceedingly painful:

If it takes much more than three minutes for them to stop hurting,

If the pain is not relieved, or partly relieved but quickly comes back again, this means the trigger points are being perpetuated either by a general excessive uptightness within yourself, or by a reaction to injury, inflammation, in the related spine joints. On either count you will need expert help.

Low neck pain

Problems coming from the low neck joints may be more severe and debilitating, and may involve a marked reaction to injury, inflammation. This is called cervical spondylitis and the condition which may provoke it (page 79) has already been described. The pain is characterized by its severity and persistence. As with the pain from a ruptured disc, there is difficulty sleeping. The sufferer wakes after only an hour or so, and then has great difficulty getting back to sleep. The pain is severe first thing in the morning and takes at least an hour or so to ease off. There is a constant nagging discomfort throughout the day which gets worse in the evening.

The pain may start behind the shoulder. In a few hours it spreads up the back of the neck, out to the shoulder, and then down the arm, often as far as the fingers and/or the thumb.

Pain down the arm may have its origin from joints higher up in the neck. Such pain relates to the development of hot trigger points in some of the shoulder girdle muscles. Remember, these muscles get their nerve supply from the neck segments of the spine.

It is important to be able to distinguish between the two types of arm pain because they need to be dealt with in two completely different ways: *Pain from a cervical spondylitis* usually spreads down the arm in a few hours or a day or so after the onset of neck pain. *Trigger point pain* may take a week or so after the onset of neck pain before spreading down the arm. It may first spread to the shoulder, then a few days later to the upper arm, then a few days later to the forearm and hand.

Trigger point pain is less severe, more patchy and less well defined. All movements of the neck and shoulder, particularly looking upwards and towards the painful side, tend to hurt in spondylitis. Muscle trigger point pain is aggravated just when the particular muscle is used: more the shoulder than the neck.

The essence of treatment for spondylitis is rest of the injured inflamed neck joints, painkillers and patience. Any active treatment, with the possible exception of simple neck traction, getting hung, will run the risk of aggravating the inflammation. Rest may be achieved with the aid of a collar; one made of sorbo-rubber is usually enough. In more severe cases a moulded stiffer collar may help. This must hold the neck in a relaxed position, the so-called high occiput (back of the head) chin tuck-in position, so that the openings at the side of the spine are as wide as possible. A rigid collar should not be kept on for too long: the rich supply of sensing nerves round the neck joints needs to be constantly stimulated, otherwise the nerves will fade away and die. Such a collar needs to be fitted by an expert, usually found in hospital surgical appliances departments. You can make your own sorbo-rubber collar. Don't forget it needs to be a quarter higher at the back than the front.

Even in cervical spondylitis the muscles round the shoulder

usually develop hot trigger points, but it is a waste of time having a go at these before the joint inflammation has settled. Once this has happened, which may take up to two months, depending on severity, local treatment to the trigger points will hasten recovery. This stage is usually signalled by a lessening of the severe pain, less disturbed sleep, and a shortening of the time it is very sore when first getting up.

If you get someone to have a go at the trigger points and they hurt too much and do not stop hurting within about three minutes, you will know there is still some reaction to injury taking place. Either that or the ongoing pain has created a lot of general uptightness. The best indication of this is continued poor quality sleep.

Long term management of this problem will be covered in the chapter on exercises and exercising.

Pains in the chest

So often one has seen people panic-stricken by a pain in the front of the chest. The immediate thought is, 'Is it my heart?' We only have one heart, and the idea that anything might be wrong with it creates panic in the stoutest. Pain in the front of the chest *may* come from a heart problem, a coronary thrombosis or angina, but it may also come from a simple problem in the neck or thoracic (chest) spine.

An overstressed joint in the mid part of the thoracic spine may lead to a pain at the front of the chest. The spread to the front is associated with the development of hot trigger points in the muscles at the side of the spine and often in the small muscles between each rib.

An overstressed neck joint may also lead to pain at the front of the chest by way of hot trigger points in some of the neck muscles and in particular the pectoral muscles.

We are more conscious of our fronts than our backs, they are more vulnerable, so a pain in the front of the chest may mask the associated sore neck or thoracic spine.

So, if you have a pain in the front of your chest, before pressing the panic button, ask yourself the following questions:

Is the pain crushing or vice-like in quality? Heart.

Or does it seem more on the surface and not so severe? Muscle trigger-point pain.

Is it relieved by moving about? Muscle.

If it wakes you in the night is it relieved by getting up and moving about, or by getting into a more comfortable position in bed? Muscle.

Is it provoked by all strenuous activity and by walking some distance, and quickly relieved by rest? Heart.

Is it just provoked by some activities, such as reaching up or twisting? Muscle.

If there is any doubt, and there must always be some, you should have your heart checked out. If your doctor's checks show there is no heart problem you may be assured nothing serious is going on, and the offending trigger points should be looked for. A word of warning: if you have a painful heart attack hot trigger points will be found in the pectoral muscles. Before local treatment to these is started the heart must be checked out.

Treatment of these trigger points with injections of local anaesthetics will in fact give relief to the pain coming from your heart, but this will not benefit the underlying heart problem.

Headaches

We all suffer headaches at some time or other: when we have a cold, a sinus infection, a hangover, and so on. Very rarely, a severe headache may be a symptom of something serious going on inside the head, such as a growth. Incidentally, it is rarely a symptom of raised blood pressure, unless this is a sudden and marked rise.

Most recurrent headaches are related to tension in the muscles at the back of the neck, provoking 'hot' painful trigger points. This local tension is in part a response to some increased wear and tear in the upper neck joints, in part a response to continued bad posture, and possibly also in part a response to life's stresses.

When standing up in a relaxed posture the body's centre of gravity passes down in a vertical line from just behind the ear.

In this position there is an equal body weight in front and behind the vertical line. We are balanced. Very little muscle activity is needed to maintain this position.

When the head is held forward, as when bending over a flat-topped desk, the weight of the head is in front of this centre of gravity. To maintain this position and to stop the head falling further forward the muscles at the back of the neck have to work continuously. They become fatigued, and there is an accumulation of waste products from overactivity. These muscles invariably contain latent trigger points, which are easily provoked by overstrain into 'hot' painful ones. The pain from these trigger points may be experienced in various parts of the head.

A common pattern of these trigger-point headaches is as follows. First there is an ache in the back of the neck. As the day passes a dull ache in the back of the head is felt. This may then spread to the front of the head to behind one or both eyes. Sometimes the spread is into the face or jaws. The sufferer may think it is toothache. Some people have lost healthy teeth because of it.

Many such recurring headaches have been labelled as tension headaches. The victim is handed a pocket full of tranquillizers and told not to worry. This is only part of the story: much more can be done.

Before going further it is necessary to distinguish this type of headache from migraine. Often people call their headaches migraine when in fact they are not.

Real *migraine* is a headache coming from local spasm of blood vessels on the surface of the brain. There is a strong inheritance factor. The migraine may be provoked by stress but other factors also play a part.

The onset of an attack of migraine may be heralded by odd visual effects, such as zig-zag lines in front of the eye, or by a feeling of numbness in part of the face, and many other odd sensations. The onset of the headache is often quite sudden, usually starting in the same place each time, such as behind one eye. Characteristically, the headache is severe and has a throb-

bing quality, pulsing with the heart beat. Usually the headache
is associated with nausea and often vomiting. Any bright light
hurts the eyes – a bed in a darkened room is the best place to
be. The attacks may last from a few hours to a day or two.
When the headache goes the victim is often left with a feeling
of fatigue. The attacks tend to recur at regular intervals.

On the other hand, *trigger point headaches* start gradually.
They are not heralded by any odd visual or other signals. There
is a constant steady ache. At times this may become sharp. There
may be some nausea but this is rare. They may only last for a
few hours and be gone after a night's sleep, or they may go on
for days and days.

When working out what can be done for these headaches the
following factors need to be considered:

Do you wake up with the headache and does it pass off after
you have been up and about for some time?

If so, a change of pillow may help. On the whole, rubber chip
pillows are not the best: there is too much bounce in them,
which does not allow the neck muscles to relax sufficiently. The
old fashioned kapok pillows are still the best: it is possible to
punch them into a shape which they will stay in. (Of course, if
you are allergic to kapok they are not a good idea.) Whether a
thick or a thin pillow is best for you depends on the shape of
your head and neck; to find the right height may need some
trial and error. Tying a piece of cord round the 'waist' of the
pillow, giving it two butterfly wings, may help. The head will
rest comfortably between the two wings.

Waking with a headache may also mean you are not relaxing
properly in your sleep. This means an overactive alerting system.
You need to ask yourself: Has my sleep pattern changed? Am
I waking earlier? Am I waking in the night where I did not
before? Ask your partner: am I tossing and turning in my sleep
more than I used to?

If the cap fits a change of pillow will not be of much help. It
is necessary to have a long careful look at the factors which
may be overstressing your coping system.

Are you waking up pain-free, the headaches coming on during

the day? If so, which days of the week? Is it during the working week or just at the weekends? If the headaches just occur at the weekends, unless you are doing something like playing a violin all weekend and not during the week, this usually means there is a source of undue stress at home.

A headache coming on during the day signifies a build-up of tension in the neck muscles. This may be due to prolonged neck flexion, or continued uptightness due to stresses in the workplace: too heavy a workload, job insecurity, boredom with the work, personality clashes with others at work, and so on. Eye-strain may play an indirect part. It is not the eyes which cause such headaches but the subconcious tension created in the neck muscles when straining all the time to see properly.

It is often said: so-and-so has bad posture. What do we mean by good or bad posture?

The ideal posture has been defined as that which can be maintained most effortlessly throughout the activities of daily living. In other words this has nothing to do with the shape we are in when we are standing up straight. There is no ideal static postural shape. We all come in different shapes and sizes. The posture we assume when standing or sitting more often reflects the image of ourselves which we wish to project to those around us: 'Look at me with my sagging shoulders and hang-dog head. Coping with all my troubles is really too much. Do have sympathy for my lot in life.' Or, 'Look at me with my chin thrust forward. I'm aggressive; don't stand in my way.' And so on.

A good posture really means one which is alert, active, and does not stay in one place too long.

As far as the neck is concerned there is one bad posture: where the head is carried well in front of the centre of gravity. In such a posture there is an increased forward curve to the neck. More of the weight of the head is in front of the centre of gravity and so the muscles in the back of the neck have to work continuously to prevent the head falling further forward. Such a posture also jams the facet joints together and they have to carry extra weight.

This posture is at least partly assumed and has become a habit – therefore to some extent it can be corrected. This will require a lot of effort over a long period of time. It is always difficult altering a bad habit, but this exercise will help to sort the problem out.

Neck stretch exercise   There is a tight band, called the ligamentum nuchae, which goes from the middle of the back of the skull down to the backward projecting spine of the lowest neck vertebra. With an increased forward curve in the neck this ligament will be slack and you will not be able to feel it with your own fingers. Also, the increased curve will cause the muscles in the back of the neck to be shortened and tight.

To flatten out this curve, thus stretching the muscles, tightening the ligament, and bringing the head back to the correct position in relation to the centre of gravity, it is necessary to make a conscious effort to push the whole head backwards, at the same time keeping the chin tucked in. To further tighten the ligament and stretch the muscles it is now necessary to sense a lifting up of the back of the head. This is the hard part. Place the fingers of one hand down the middle of the back of the neck, so that you will be able to feel the tightening of the ligament. Now try to consciously elevate the back of the head. As you get the hang of lifting up the back of the head you will feel this central ligament tighten up.

Once you have got into this position it should be held for about ten to fifteen seconds, and then relaxed. It should be repeated four or five times, and it should be done as often as you can remember throughout the day. If you are sitting at a desk most of the day or driving a car for long distances this exercise should be repeated at about fifteen-minute intervals. Apart from noticing you have developed an extra chin or two no one will think any the worse of you for doing it.

There really is a need for the habit of correct neck and head posture to be instilled into us at an early age, at home and at school. It is so easy to get into this bad posture, with the head carried well in front of the centre of gravity. Once our computers have become programmed into holding this position it is the devil's own job to break the habit.

If you work sitting at a desk or a machine all day it is important to pay careful attention to your position.

Is your seat at the right height in relation to the desk top? Has the seat an adequate back rest, fitting into the small of your back, so that you can sit up straight and feel comfortable? Is the machine you are working at the right height so that you do not have to bend your neck forward continually?

From what has been written earlier you will have gathered there is no such thing as an ideal chair. In fact it could be said the more comfortable the chair the more likely one is to sit in it for too long. In a perfect world, all those working in a sitting position would stand up every fifteen minutes or so and do a minute of simple calisthenics. The lost work time would be more than compensated by increased efficiency and less time off work because of sore necks and backs.

If you are plagued by these postural stress headaches, wearing a light collar for a time may be a help. A home-made one cut out of a piece of thick sorbo-rubber and covered with some stockinette will be adequate. Remember, it should be a quarter higher at the back than the front. Most of these collars which are available on the market are designed so they fasten at the back, but if you do this most of them are higher at the front, so you have to reverse them and fasten them under your chin. Someone is bound to come up and tell you your collar is the wrong way round. You can assure them this is not so.

Wearing such a collar at work will have side benefits: it will evoke sympathy in your fellow workers.

Such a collar may be very useful to have in your car. It may save you from a sore neck and headache on a long car journey.

The fact that you are prone to these headaches means there is some wear and tear in the joints of the upper part of your neck. Putting increased strain on these joints will lead to reflex tightening in the muscles, and thus possibly convert a latent trigger point into a 'hot' painful one. Nothing can be done about the wear and tear so any preventative strategy has to be ongoing.

The exercises and posture correction have to be maintained indefinitely.

There is one other muscle which tends to get tight when we get uptight and when we are working over a desk with hunched shoulders and forward thrusting neck. Trigger points in this muscle, known as the trapezius muscle, are a common source of headaches.

The trapezius muscle is attached to the side of the spine from the base of the skull right down to the lower part of the thoracic spine (see Fig. 47). It is inserted mainly into the upper inner edge of the shoulder blade, and is thus fan shaped.

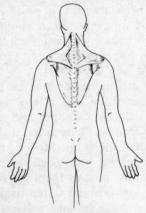

Figure 47 *The upper and lower trapezius muscle*

When working together on both sides, the muscle fibres coming from the neck pull the shoulder blade up and also increase the forward curve of the neck. If we are already in this position these muscle fibres will tend to stay short and tight. Therefore, frequent stretches to the upper part of the trapezius as well as to the other muscles in the back of the neck will help to prevent postural stress headaches. This is how you do it:

Upper trapezius stretch exercise   Sit upright in a chair which has no arms. If you wish to stretch the right upper trapezius

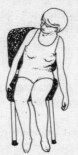

Figure 48 *The upper trapezius muscle stretch*

muscle grasp the bottom of the seat with your right hand, level with your hip joint (see Fig. 48). Now bend your head half way forward. Then side bend it to the left. Then twist it to the right so that you are looking down on your right hand. Now side bend your whole trunk to the left. As you do this you will feel this muscle tighten in the back of your neck. When you feel a tightness stop in that position. Now, without moving any part of your head or body, pull up hard with your right hand. This will make the muscle contract whilst in a stretched position. Keep pulling for a slow count of seven, about seven seconds. Then relax the pull and immediately bend the trunk further to the left without altering the relative position of your head. This will further take up any slack in the muscle which was gained by the resisted contraction. In the new position now repeat the pull with the right hand for a further seven seconds. The interval between each pull should be as short as possible, about three seconds, not more. Three stretches and three pulls are all that is required, so it does not take long.

This exercise, like the neck stretch, cannot be overdone. It should be understood that it may help you but only for as long as you keep on doing it.

Partial deafness Before leaving these common tension headaches it is worth mentioning that those who are partially deaf are particularly prone to them. In order to try and hear better it becomes a habit to thrust the head forward, in front of the centre of gravity. This results in continuous activity in the muscles at the back of the neck. This, combined with the tension created by the effort of trying to hear, may easily provoke painful muscle spasm.

Headache trigger points   If you are prone to these tension headaches it is worth knowing where to look for the 'hot' trigger points.

One is usually found just below the back of the skull, on one or both sides of the back of the neck spine. Another is usually to be found just above the inner upper angle of the shoulder blade. (See Fig. 49.) It is possible to get at these yourself. To do so you must first relax your head and neck, either by resting back in a comfortable chair with your head supported, or by lying on your back with your head resting on a thick pillow.

To feel for the trigger points, use the hand on the opposite side. Hook the middle finger and use it to poke hard into the muscles just to the side of the mid line. Move the finger from side to side. Start just under the back of the skull and slowly work down. There is no mistaking the trigger point: there is

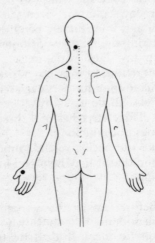

Figure 49 *Common headache trigger points*

marked local tenderness. Press hard and keep the pressure up until it stops hurting.

To locate the one near the upper inner angle of the shoulder blade, reach across the front of the chest. It is easy to locate the angle of the shoulder blade on the opposite side. Again using the hooked middle finger, poke hard into the muscle just above this angle and slightly nearer to the spine. Poke around until the trigger point is located, and then maintain firm pressure until it stops hurting.

If you find this too difficult to do yourself, get someone else to have a go. If their fingers are not strong enough apply the pressure with something which has a blunt end. The old fashioned flat topped wooden clothes peg is ideal. A bit of extra padding may be fastened over the end.

There is one other common 'hot' trigger point often associated with recurrent headaches. This can be found in the muscles in the web between the thumb and first finger. Why this particular trigger point should get 'hot' when we get a headache is not known, but it is a traditional Chinese acupuncture point for headaches. Perhaps there are other trigger points which get 'hot' when we get uptight enough to provoke a headache, which in the past have not been looked for.

This trigger point is very easy to get at and can very easily be pressured by trapping it between the first finger and thumb of the opposite hand.

It is necessary to get at these trigger points before the headache has become firmly established. Immediately after pressuring the trigger points it is then necessary to stretch out the muscles by using the two exercises which have been described.

If the headache has become firmly established the trigger points will be found to be too 'hot' and tender and will not go away by pressuring. If this has happened the only thing to do is put up with it, take two or three aspirins, and lie down, if possible.

Alternative treatment   Physical treatment such as manipulation and acupuncture usually have little of value to offer in the overall management of tension headaches. They may give temporary relief and may be used with this in mind, but they are no replacement for the understanding and necessary counter-measures required for the postural and stress factors.

If there is a one-off attack of neck pain and headache due to a physical overstress of worn neck joints, such treatment may give rapid relief. This may be all the treatment necessary, but if there are frequent recurrences such local treatment should be abandoned. No lasting benefit will accrue, and the real source of the problem is being ignored.

Treatment of whiplash injuries

Whiplash injuries can cause much pain and suffering, but with proper rest and carefully-timed treatment, a good deal can be done to alleviate pain and speed the healing process.

If the accident was severe and there was almost immediate noticeable neck pain an X-ray, to exclude possible bone damage, will be necessary. If the X-ray shows no damage, that will be reassuring, but remember, X-rays cannot show soft tissue damage, such as a ligament or joint capsule sprain. If noticeable discomfort does not develop until the next day or so an X-ray, except for reassurance purposes, will be of little value.

Even if the accident was minor there may have been some soft tissue damage. This should have led to some immediate discomfort which may not have become noticeable till a few hours later, or even when first waking up the next day.

If there is tissue damage, however minor, the only logical treatment is rest of the injured part. A light sorbo-rubber collar may help. A rigid collar, for reasons already given (page 142), is to be avoided if possible.

The question of how long the collar should be worn is important. Most minor soft tissue strains and sprains should be healed in about two weeks, so this should be a sufficient time to be wearing a collar. It can easily become a habit if you wear it for longer.

In the presence of healing tissue no active treatment, such as manipulation, will be of any help. Stimulation of the pain nerves by the reaction to injury usually reflexly provokes potentially self-perpetuating painful trigger points. It is of no value to have a go at these triggers until the reaction to injury is over and done with.

After about two weeks the pain should have subsided and now become more off and on, just provoked by certain movements, not unduly disturbing sleep, and quickly easing off after getting out of bed. Now is the time to try local treatment. Manipulation and/or trigger point treatment may be tried. If this does not give rapid relief or seems to aggravate the pain it means either the reaction to injury is still going on or an over-active alerting system has become a nuisance. In either case, local treatment should be immediately abandoned. Any local treatment should be combined with the two stretch exercises which have been described (pages 148 and 150–151).

Acute wry neck

With no noticeable prior warning some people have the misfortune to wake up in the night or first thing in the morning with a very stiff and painful neck. It is difficult to get the head off the pillow and the slightest movement is very painful. The head is held in the side bend position; hence the name. Such attacks mainly afflict people in their late teens and early twenties; they are more common in those who have naturally very mobile necks.

What probably happens can only be speculation, but the fact that the side bend of the neck is usually away from the side which is painful, suggests that something painful has become trapped between the surfaces of the facet joints. This is probably one of the little meniscoids which carry a rich supply of pain nerve endings.

The best first aid treatment is to apply an ice pack: a packet of frozen peas wrapped in some thin towelling will do, kept against the back of the neck for about twenty minutes at a time. Some aspirin or equivalent may be needed.

The possible value of any other active treatment is debatable. Should you go to a manipulator? Those who manipulate, myself included, feel that help can be given. If something is trapped, freeing this entrapment should solve the problem and relieve the severe pain. Any attempt to do this requires great care; it is so easy to provoke further painful muscle spasm. To prise open the facet joints where the supposed entrapment is requires a gradual increase in the side bend already present combined with some carefully applied traction to the neck. If this is done carefully you should not suffer undue discomfort. There should be some immediate relief, but it still takes two or three days for all the painful spasm to settle.

There is also some evidence to suggest that most attacks, even if nothing is done, will settle in two to three days. So, you have a choice. It would certainly be cheaper to stay at home and rest. Certainly, if there is no improvement after three days, a visit to a manipulator could be worth while. Remember, if manipulation is going to help it will do so quickly.

Treatment of stress overload

By now you will have understood how getting uptight may in part be responsible for the onset of a sore neck or back. If you did not start by being uptight the sore neck or back is eventually likely to make you so. Being uptight is certainly in large part responsible for a neck or back pain keeping on when it should have disappeared.

It is a very difficult task to try and persuade people that their back or neck keeps on hurting because they are too uptight. They will feel that you are suggesting they are neurotic, non-coping individuals. This is far from the truth. It is not that we are not coping but that the effort involved in coping is having the effect of making our muscles too uptight.

As already mentioned (pages 104–105), we have a built-in ability to cope, which shows a wide variation from individual to individual. How much this individual coping ability is due to genetic factors and how much due to early environmental factors is debatable, but however good or bad we are at coping we may all become overloaded. When we are overloaded our primitive alerting system becomes overactive. This is when we start to get into trouble.

If we take the threshold of coping overload as a horizontal line most of us drift through life below this line, some of us nearer to it than others. When increased stress is imposed on us we may cross this threshold line. Then problems arise. So, you say, 'What can you do for my uptightness, Doctor?' The simple answer is: very little. I cannot alter the environmental factors responsible for you being in overload. Anyway, I'm no expert on stress management. I have enough trouble coping with my own problems.

'Then who should I go to?'

Well, your own family doctor may be able to help. There is an increasing awareness of how stress overloads may cause or aggravate various medical problems. Some family doctors have taken up what is called 'counselling'. You unload your problems into a sympathetic, non-judgemental ear. This may result in some temporary release of tension, but talking about what has happened in the past will not alter it, and talking about the shortcomings of others around you is not going to alter them. Understanding why you react to stresses the way you do does not necessarily mean you can alter that reaction. You will not be given any positive advice, told what to do. This is too dangerous. If you followed such advice and things went wrong the person giving the advice could be held responsible.

It is unlikely a psychiatrist would be much help to you. They are trained to help those considered by society to be mentally abnormal. There is nothing abnormal about this problem. Psychologists have taken over the mantle of the expert in the field of stress management. Here again, one could question their ability to alter you or your environment significantly.

The response to overstress is manifested as an increase in aggression, or the opposite, regression, or somewhere between the two. The response is anger, fear, anxiety, depending on the stimulus. We are a naturally aggressive species. The only other species capable of deliberately killing those of the same kind are rats (discount certain female insects who gobble up their mates). This aggression has to be understood and controlled for there to be hope of species survival. Some psychologists run classes to teach people how to cope with stress and anger: let it out; don't bottle it up.

Such advice may have its drawbacks: you may end up with no friends at all.

Stress may be reduced by tricks such as transcendental meditation, self-hypnosis, relaxation exercises. All worth a go. What stress overload really adds up to, which should be a comfort to the sufferer, is that the problem is not really within the individual but in the society in which he or she lives. There is not a lot the individual can do about that.

Having said this, it is still possible for the individual to help him or herself, without resource to potentially expensive outside agencies. We are designed to respond to incoming sensations by action, motion, using our muscles. Failure to respond to incoming sensations by action creates tension within the individual. Basically we move towards pleasant sensations and away from the unpleasant.

A continuing programme of vigorous exercise is a practical solution. By all means understand the reasons why you are overstressed, practise transcendental meditation, relaxation exercises, yoga, and so on, but also shift yourself!

How to go about a vigorous exercise programme will be explained in the chapter on exercise.

Perhaps a punch-bag in the garage may help, with the face of the main source of overstress painted on the bag, as long as it is not one of the family. Don't kick the cat.

Prevention

Exercises

So, you have recovered from your attack of neck or back pain. By now you should understand, from whatever help you have or have not received, you are not cured. The fact that you have had this attack tells you there is some wear and tear in your spine. It should also be understood that uptight irritable muscles have played some part in the attack.

You will now be able to see that there is a need for plenty of movement to prevent further premature ageing of the spinal joints. So you wish to know if there are specific exercises which can be done to prevent recurrences. Yes, there are, as long as they continue to be done.

The question is: what exercises?

Some experts recommend flexion compliance exercises — exercises designed to make it easier to bend without unduly stressing the spine. This is all very well in theory, but allowing such continued flexion of the spine would put the back wall of the disc at risk. This is all right if the disc is young and healthy, but if there is premature wear and tear such exercises can be hazardous.

Other experts recommend the opposite: frequent bending back of the spine. This is good because it relaxes all the ligaments and muscles behind the pivot point, the disc nucleus, thus preventing painful overstretching of the ligaments and fatigue in the muscles due to continuous forward bending of the spine. Such bending backwards will also tend to squeeze forward any fragments of worn disc nucleus, helping to keep them out of harm's way. But it has the disadvantage of further jamming the low back facet joints into each other. These may already be vulnerable from associated disc narrowing and wear and tear.

Some experts recommend back strengthening exercises, raising the head and chest from the lying prone position. From what has been written in the section on the muscles (pages 40–45) you will realize the back muscles are not designed as strength muscles but for speed of action and range of motion; and because they are close to the pivot of movement, they are not efficient strength muscles. Also, they are classified as postural muscles which tend to get short and tight without any further help. Increasing the strength of these muscles will tend to increase the load on the low back facet joints which may already be compromised from previous wear and tear.

Abdominal muscles

It is generally agreed the abdominal muscles should be strengthened. There is no doubt strength in these muscles helps to unload the strain on our spines when we do any lifting. These muscles are called phasic. This means they come into action mainly when we are on the go. They are used hardly at all when we are sitting. Putting your hand on your own stomach now, while you are sitting reading, will confirm this fact: the muscles feel soft and flabby.

Muscles which are not being used quickly become weak. If you look around at your fellow beings out in the street, you will quickly see just how weak and flabby the abdominal muscles may become.

The abdominal muscles are a long way from the pivot point of movement in the spine. Their action whilst lifting therefore protects and buffers the spinal joints. Imagine a seesaw, the pivot point of the seesaw being the disc nucleus (see Fig. 50). To lift a weight at one end of the seesaw just by using the muscles close to the pivot point on the other end (the back muscles) would require tremendous effort by the muscles and would impose a tremendous load on the discs. If you now interpose a strong loaded spring (the abdominal muscles), and between that and the pivot point an enclosed tense bag (the

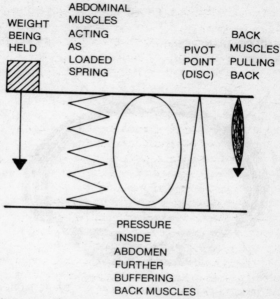

Figure 50 *The human see-saw pivoting round the disc:* The back muscles were not designed for strength. They are too near the pivot point. The strength for lifting is provided by strong rump, thigh, leg, and abdominal muscles. Strong abdominals convert the abdomen into a rigid tube. This unloads the pivot point, the disc, and takes the stress off the back muscles.

abdominal cavity), you can see how this will reduce the compression loading of the spine and reduce the effort needed by the back muscles.

The abdominal muscles at the front, called the rectus abdominus, have muscle fibres which run straight up and down. When they contract they pull the spine forwards, or conversely, resist the spine from being pulled backwards.

Around the sides of the abdomen is a layer of three other muscles. The outer two of these have muscle fibres which run obliquely to those of the front muscle, the rectus abdominus (see Fig. 51). The inner muscle has fibres which run at right angles to the rectus. The outer two muscles assist the front muscle to pull the trunk forward. They also assist or resist

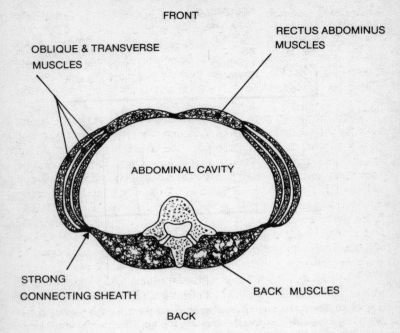

Figure 51 *Cross section of the abdominal and back muscles:* The abdominal and back muscles are surrounded by a strong connecting fibrous sheath. In the flank the fibres of this sheath run in a criss-cross fashion. This gives them added strength. When the abdominal muscles are strong and contract they exert tension on the sheath surrounding the back muscles, thus helping to make them more effective.

twisting of the trunk. All three also resist sideways bulging of the abdomen, thus helping to increase the pressure inside the abdomen. All the abdominal muscles when working together have a further important function. They are all surrounded by a very strong sheath which is connected to the sheath surrounding the main back muscles. When these abdominal muscles contract they put tension on this sheath. This will increase the tension on the back muscles and therefore help them to be more effective when they contract.

Abdominal muscle strengthening exercise A frequently prescribed abdominal strengthening exercise is as follows:

Lie on your back with the knees and hips bent (called the crook lying position). Lock your hands behind your head. From this position sit up, trying to bring your nose to your knees. There are variations of this which also impose a twist to one side or the other.

There is one snag to this exercise. If you place your hands over the front of the pelvis of someone who is doing the exercise you will find that after the first ten degrees or so of sitting up the pelvis will begin to rotate forwards. The contracting abdominal muscles should continue to pull the pelvis the other way, so this means there must be some other muscle coming into the action. There is – the iliopsoas muscle which has already been described (pages 129–130). This may already be shortened and tight; it is an important postural muscle, so such an exercise will tend to make it shorter and tighter still. This may make the problem worse.

If you feel a strong urge to strengthen your abdominal muscles this is how you should do it (see Fig. 52). From the crook lying position, lying on your back with the knees and hips bent, lift your shoulders just off the floor and stop there. At the same time, push down hard with your feet, and press back towards yourself with your heels. This will relax the iliopsoas muscle.

A word of warning. Abdominal strengthening exercises dramatically increase the pressure inside the low back discs. If these are weakened from previous wear and tear such exercises are best avoided.

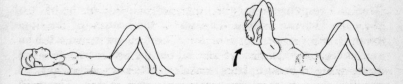

Figure 52 *Abdominal muscle strengthening exercise:* Do not go further than just raising the shoulders off the ground.

Calf muscles

When planning an exercise programme the following principles, based on research by Professor Vladimir Janda from Prague, should be followed: First, tight postural muscles should be stretched out. When these are stretched out strengthening exercises for the phasic muscles may be used, but not before.

It is therefore necessary to determine which of your postural muscles are tight. It would be a waste of time stretching out muscles which don't need to be stretched. This is why a universal set programme of exercises may waste a lot of time. An exercise programme needs to be tailored to individual requirements.

To start with, we should look for tight muscles which may be affecting our ability to bend with the minimum stress on the spine. This means bending with the hips and knees, not the back. You should be able to squat down with the feet staying flat on the ground. If you cannot do this without tipping over backwards it means you have tight muscles in the back of your calf which are preventing you from bending forward at the ankle, in order to keep your weight over your flat feet. More about this in a moment.

The muscle responsible for restricting the ability to bend forward at the ankle, with the knees also bent, is called the soleus muscle. This lies in the middle of the back of the calf. It arises from the back of the two leg bones just below the knee. At the ankle it becomes part of the thick tendon (the achilles) attached to the heel bone. When it contracts it pulls up the back of the ankle, thus pulling the forefoot down.

There are two other muscles, called the gastrocnaemiae, which make up the rest of the attachment into the achilles tendon. They are responsible for the bulge on each side of the back of the calf. They arise from the back of the bottom of the thigh bone (femur). They cross the knee joint. Thus, when we bend our knees these muscles are relaxed but the soleus muscle is not. If we wish to bend up the foot when the knee is straight it is mainly the gastrocnaemiae which restrict the movement. Bending the foot up with the knee bent is restricted by the soleus muscle. Thus, the ability to squat comfortably depends on the soleus, while tightness in the achilles tendon when walking and running is due to the gastrocnaemiae. Such tightness is responsible for achilles tendon problems in runners. It is easy to pick out people who suffer from it if you watch them walking: the heel of the back leg as they take a step is picked off the ground early. These muscles are prone to night cramps as we get older, and regular stretching is a better way of preventing them than taking drugs.

Here, as promised, is how to test for tightness in these two muscles.

Test for gastroc-soleus tightness While lying on your back with the legs straight out ask someone to push your foot back towards you. The foot should be pushed back from near the ankle, otherwise the bending backwards of the forefoot may give a false idea of how much bending there is at the ankle joint. The foot should come back about ten degrees past the vertical.

However, the ability to squat comfortably with the feet remaining flat on the ground is still the best test.

Gastroc-soleus stretch exercise First, the principles of stretch exercises should be restated: muscles may be stretched out by applying a slow steady stretch, applied for about fifteen seconds at a time and repeated ten to fifteen times; or by using the hold-relax technique. Hold-relax takes less time, but they are both about equally effective. One should not attempt to stretch a muscle by using a bouncing action – this is likely to do more harm than good.

Muscles will not stretch out if

1   there is still some reaction to injury in the associated spinal joints.
2   there are still hot trigger points in the muscle or associated muscles sharing a common nerve supply.
3   the owner of the muscle is too uptight.

So, as with all exercises, if it hurts – stop. Try again another day. The idea that one has to suffer pain in order to get better is ingrained in many minds. It is not true that you have to go through hell in order to reach heaven.

It should also be understood that if a muscle has become tight it is likely to get tight again. This applies particularly to those muscles which are kept in a shortened position for too long, as happens with prolonged sitting. This applies to the gastrocsoleus muscles. So, to remain effective, any stretching has to be continued ad infinitum unless the pattern of everyday living is altered.

Stand facing a wall. Rest the outstretched hands against the wall. Bend one leg forward at the hip and knee. Slide the other leg backwards, keeping the knee straight. The foot of this backward leg should be kept turned slightly inwards (see Fig. 53). As the leg slides further backwards a tightness in the calf will be felt. Stop at this point. From this position, keeping the body and legs still, push down hard with the foot of the backward leg. Keep this push going for a slow count of seven (about seven seconds) and then relax. Immediately put more stretch on the muscle by allowing the elbows to bend and the body to go forward. Keep the same alignment of the body to the backward leg: do not allow the trunk to cave in. As soon as the muscle feels tight again, stop. Then repeat the downward push of the

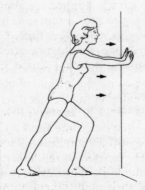

Figure 53 *Calf muscle stretch:* Keep the back foot slightly turned in. If you allow the low back to cave in this will also stretch the iliopsoas muscle. If this is also tight the exercise will serve a dual purpose.

foot. The relaxing stretching interval should be as short as possible — about three seconds.

This procedure should be repeated three times and end up
with a final stretch.

The stretch in these muscles may be maintained by taking up
the increasingly unpopular pastime of walking. A regular long
walk, deliberately striding out, would obviate the need for
prolonged stretching exercises. Frequent squatting will have the
same beneficial effect.

Hamstring muscles

Another group of postural muscles which frequently get short
and tight are those known as the hamstrings. They consist of
three muscles, two on one side and one on the other, in the
back of the thigh. They arise from a promontory on the back
of the pelvis, and are inserted into the main bone of the leg
(tibia) just below the knee. Therefore, they cross two joints, the
hip and the knee.

When the muscles contract a pull will be imposed on the back
of the pelvis, pulling it downwards and backwards as it pivots
round the hip joint. A pull on the other end will bend the knee
and pull the leg backwards.

In four-legged animals these muscles have the important function of allowing the animal to rear up on its hind legs. Having
reared up on our hind legs and stayed there, and because of the
changed shape of the pelvis, the origin of these muscles has
moved nearer to the joint they move (see Fig. 54). They have
therefore become a less efficient mover of the hip joint. The
rump muscles (gluteals) have become the important backward
benders of the hips. The upright stance has straightened out our
knees. To allow this the insertion of the hamstring muscles has
had to move closer to the knee. They are no longer an efficient
bender of the knee, and their main function now is to maintain
the upright stance, by stopping the hips bending. Most times,
gravity will do the bending for us.

Thus the hamstrings are not very efficient movers of either

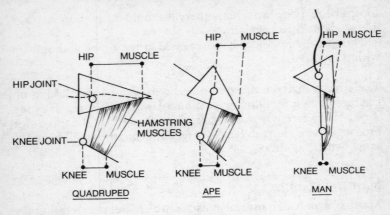

Figure 54 *The evolution of the hamstring muscles:* In arriving at the upright stance, the origin of the muscle becomes closer to the hip joint, and the insertion to the knee joint.

the hips or the knees. In fact, they have become a bit of a nuisance. In battles of long ago, soldiers taken prisoner on the field of battle used to have the tendons of these muscles cut with a sword, or similar weapon. This stopped them in their tracks and reduced their chances of running away. They could be picked up later when the battle was over, and were still mobile enough to act as efficient slaves. Hence the expression, 'being hamstrung'.

When we bend forward with our knees straight we should be able to pivot round our hips about 80 to 90 degrees. This brings the trunk more or less horizontal to the ground. Taking into account the length of the arms, this means very little bending of the spine will be necessary to pick something up from ground level. When the hamstrings are tight this ability to pivot round the hips will be reduced. They act as struts, limiting the upward movement of the back of the pelvis as it rotates round the hips (see Fig. 55). This means the spine has to be bent more when picking things off the floor.

When the hamstrings are tight the ability to stride out when

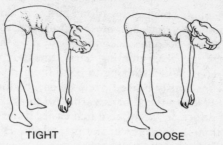

TIGHT   LOOSE

Figure 55 *The effect on bending of tight and loose hamstrings*

walking is reduced: the front leg becomes restricted in how far forward it will swing. Trying to force a long stride will make the pelvis swing round, thus imposing a twisting stress on the spine. This will be even more marked when running.

It is difficult to test how much stretch there is in your own hamstrings, but it is easy to see who has and who has not got tight hamstrings by looking at them from the side when they bend to touch their toes with the knees straight. Those with tight hamstrings do a lot of the bending with their spines rather than the hips. The take-off angle at the base of the spine remains more vertical than it should and there is marked bowing of the spine. This puts the joints of the spine at risk.

Let me now describe a common faulty pattern of bending seen in our youngsters, especially males. When they are asked to touch their toes with the knees straight, first there is a dropping of the head and shoulders. Then the top of the spine starts to bend. This is followed by the lower spine. At the very bottom of the spine there is very little bending at all. To compensate for the loss of pivot round the hips there is more bending of the spine. In the young this is noticeable in the upper part of the low back spine. Here, and in the low chest spine, there is often some wear and tear from previous Scheuermann's Disease. Any prolonged bending when the knees cannot be fully bent may thus become very sore.

To correct this faulty pattern of bending it is first necessary to stretch out the hamstrings. Once these have stretched out it is then necessary to reprogramme the computer to bend the hips and not the spine. This can be a long and very difficult process. Once our computer has become programmed to perform any movement which becomes second nature it is the devil's own job to change the programming. First, the start of the pattern has to be altered. When starting to bend the head and shoulders have to be consciously braced back. Then, the low back has to be consciously kept arched backwards. All this takes a long time and a lot of effort. It would be much easier if the computer had been programmed properly in the first place. This falls on the shoulders of parents and teachers.

It is possible to get some idea of how tight your hamstrings are. To do this you need the help of somebody else. Here is what you do:

Lie on your back on a couch or bed, or even on the floor. Ask someone to raise one of your legs slowly, using one of their hands. While this is being done you must consciously keep the knee straight and the leg relaxed. As the leg is being raised, when the limit of stretch in the hamstrings has been reached, you will be aware of a sense of tightness in the back of the thigh. When all the stretch has been taken out of the hamstrings the muscle starts to pull the pelvis round. If the person who is raising your leg puts his or her spare hand on the front of the opposite side of your pelvis he or she will be aware of when the pelvis starts to be twisted round.

If the hamstrings are loose the leg will go up to 80 or 90 degrees before tightness is experienced. If they are very tight the leg will only go up to 30 to 40 degrees.

With practice the amount of stretch in the hamstrings can be measured very accurately. This has made it a very useful muscle for research purposes. Out of this research has come the following information:

When most people get uptight their hamstrings become shorter and tighter. This reflects the muscle's spindle sensitivity to general fusimotor nerve activity: we do not have good conscious control over this muscle's tightness. When we are uptight it is shorter and tighter. When we are more relaxed it becomes more relaxed. The muscle will thus be more vulnerable to stretching strains when we are under stress.

Youngsters, particularly males, who have had Scheuermann's Disease have relatively tight hamstrings.

Manipulation of the spine from the lower thoracic (chest) region of the spine down, and local treatment to trigger points in the muscles of the back in the same region and also in the rump muscles, will immediately, reflexly, relax the hamstring muscles. Thus the degree of tightness in the hamstrings may reflect wear and tear in the spine and also uptightness within the individual. Therefore it is a waste of time trying to stretch out these muscles if there is a reaction to injury still going on in the lower spine or if the individual is under undue stress.

Some individuals are born with naturally short tight hamstrings. They have always found it impossible to touch their toes with straight knees. This may run in families. It is a waste of time trying to stretch out such intrinsically tight muscles.

Hamstring stretch exercises There are commonly recommended exercises for stretching out the hamstrings — most of which are wrong. One correct way will be described later, but first, we will see how *not* to stretch them. A frequently prescribed exercise is to rest one foot on a horizontal bar or a table more or less level with your pelvis (see Fig. 56). Keeping

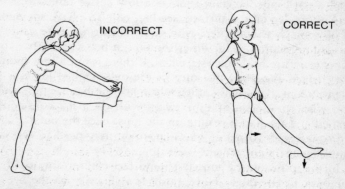

INCORRECT   CORRECT

Figure 56 *The wrong and right way to stretch the hamstrings*

the extended knee straight, you are then exhorted to reach
forward to touch the foot of the extended leg. Let's say your
hamstrings are tight and can only be raised about forty degrees
from the horizontal while you are lying on your back. If you
now stand up and raise one leg to an angle of forty degrees
from the other you will see the heel will only be about a foot
or so off the ground. To then raise the leg to a more-or-less
horizontal position will grossly overstretch the muscle. The over-
tight muscle will pull the pelvis back. To stop yourself from
falling flat on your back it will be necessary to bend forward
with your spine. To reach the outstretched foot it will be
necessary to further bend the spine. In other words, such an
exercise will be stretching the back muscles as much if not more
than the hamstrings.

This in itself may not be too bad a thing, these muscles may
be helped by a stretch, but if you also have a faulty habit of
bending, using the spine too much and the hips not enough, as
is so often the case, such a repeated exercise will tend to augment
the faulty pattern of bending.

More important, when you stretch these back muscles there
is a reflex feedback to the hamstrings via the fusimotor nerves
which will run the risk of reflexly tightening the muscle. This is
opposite to the desired effect, so let's try something better.

Find a flat-topped surface such as a low coffee table. Rest the
heel of one leg on the surface (see Fig. 56). You have some idea
of how much stretch there is in your hamstrings. The angle of
this leg in relation to the other should not be so great that your
hamstrings are being overstretched. If there is not a low enough
flat surface available, the knee of the outstretched leg may be
slightly bent. This will sufficiently relax the hamstrings which
you wish to stretch. Stand straight with the back consciously
arched and the hands resting on the hips. Face the outstretched
leg square on. To maintain balance you may need to rest one
hand against a convenient wall.

In this position the muscle should feel comfortably tight, in
the back of the thigh. Now, push down hard with the heel of
the outstretched leg for the usual slow count of seven. Then

relax and immediately slide the heel further forward on the flat surface till the muscle feels tight again. To do this it is necessary to bend the supporting back leg slightly. From this new position again push down hard with the heel. As with all these hold-relax exercises it is necessary for the relax-stretch interval to be as short as possible: not more than three seconds. Also, all these hold-relax sequences only need repeating three times, ending up with a final stretch.

Iliopsoas and rectus femoris muscles

The iliopsoas muscle has already (page 129) been described. The part of the muscle which is of most concern is that which arises from the side of the front of the low back spine. If this part is short and tight, when we are standing with our legs straight it will pull the low back spine forward, thus increasing the sway in the low back. This will also have the effect of tilting the pelvis forward round the hip joints.

The muscle is inserted into the inside front part of the upper thigh bone (femur). Sitting, with the thighs bent forward, will thus relax this end of the muscle – it will be in a shortened position. It is a postural muscle, so after prolonged sitting it will tend to get short and tight. This will have the effect of increasing the sway in the low back when standing, walking and running. This will increase the load on the low back facet joints. If the facet joints are worn and the discs are narrowed the increased stress could provoke painful muscle spasm, thus producing a posturally provoked pain after prolonged standing, walking or jogging.

The iliopsoas muscle may become short and tight on one side if there is increased wear and tear in one hip joint: the muscle shares a common nerve supply with the casing of the hip joint. This one-sided tightness will pull the low back to one side, increase the sway on one side, and also tilt the pelvis forward on one side. It will have the effect of lifting the leg on this side, leading to an apparent shortening of the leg. This results in a typical walking gait which can be recognized from a mile away. Orthopaedic surgeons may cut this muscle tendon in order to reduce the stresses it is creating. Repeated stretch exercises for this muscle will reduce the discomfort experienced from a worn hip joint.

The iliopsoas muscle is coupled with the rectus femoris muscle because they both cross the hip joint and are both capable of flexing the thigh forwards. The rectus femoris muscle is the one in the middle of the front of the thigh. This and a muscle on each side of it form the mass of muscle at the front of the thigh (quadriceps femoris muscle). It arises from a promontory on the front of the pelvis and is inserted into the knee-cap, which itself is attached to the front of the main leg bone (tibia) by means of a strong tendon.

A pull on the top end of the muscle will therefore bend the thigh forward, while a pull on the bottom end will straighten out the knee.

The rectus femoris is also in a shortened position when sitting, particularly if the knees are not fully bent, as when driving a car, so it may become shortened and tight.

If it is shortened and tight it will also tend to pull the pelvis forward round the hips when standing, thus increasing the sway in the low back. When walking and running such tightness will also restrict the backward swing of the thigh. This will have the effect of pulling the pelvis back on one side, thus causing a twist. This in turn will impose an increased twisting stress on the spine. From what has already been explained you will understand the major part of this increased twisting stress will fall on the junction of the thoracic (chest) and low back spine, so often the site of previous wear and tear.

Test for iliopsoas and rectus femoris tightness Both these muscles may be tested at the same time (see Fig. 57). Lie on your back on a firm bed or couch, with your thighs and legs hanging over the end. Grab hold of one thigh by locking both hands just below the knee. Pull this thigh back as far as it will go on to the front of your chest.

In this position, if the iliopsoas muscle is tight, the other thigh will be lifted above the horizontal line with the rest of your

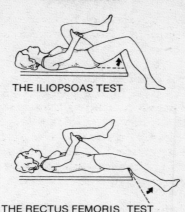

THE ILIOPSOAS TEST

THE RECTUS FEMORIS TEST

Figure 57

body. If the rectus femoris muscle is tight the thigh will be horizontal but the leg will not hang down at right angles to the thigh; it will be pulled forwards. If they are both tight the thigh will be pulled upwards by the iliopsoas and the leg will be pulled forward by the rectus femoris.

Stretches for the iliopsoas and rectus femoris muscles   One way of stretching the iliopsoas has already been described (page 130). It may also be stretched in the standing position, the so-called 'fencer's stretch'.

Get into the fencer's position, with one leg forward, the other back, and the trunk vertical (see Fig. 58). The front leg should be bent at right angles at the knee and the back leg more or less straight. The foot of the back leg should be turned slightly inwards. Remember, the muscle is attached to the inside of the top of the thigh. By turning the foot inwards it will increase the stretch on the muscle. To keep your balance, rest one hand on the forward knee and the other on your hip. If you feel unsteady one hand can rest against a convenient wall. In this position you should feel a comfortable tightness in the groin of the backward leg. Now, keeping still, push down hard with the backward foot for the usual slow count of seven. Then relax

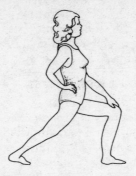

Figure 58 *The fencer's stretch*

and immediately further bend the thigh and knee of the forward
leg. Be careful to maintain a vertical, fully arched back. The
same rules apply as for other hold-relax exercises: repeat three
times, ending up with a final stretch forward.

A tight rectus femoris muscle may be stretched out in the
following way (see Fig. 59). Rest one hand on a convenient
wall. Bring one foot up behind you and grab it with the other
hand. Fully flex this knee and pull the thigh backwards until it

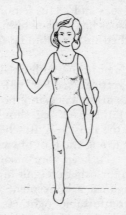

Figure 59 *The rectus femoris muscle stretch*

feels tight in the front of the thigh. Now hold the foot steady and pull hard with the foot, against the hand, for the usual seven seconds. Relax, and immediately pull the thigh further back. Repeat three times.

Hip adductor muscles

These are the muscles on the inside of the thigh which pull the knees together whenever this is necessary. Strong, well-stretched adductor muscles are necessary to horse riders, allowing a good grip with the knees when the thighs are well apart. The adductor group of muscles arise from the pubic bone at the front of the pelvis and are inserted down the length of the inside of the thigh bone. Their main action is to pull the thigh bones together. Most of them also pull the thigh forward and twist it outwards. Therefore, when sitting they will be in a shortened position, especially if the knees are crossed. Particularly in those who have to sit for long hours they may be tight. They also tend to get tight if there is wear and tear in the hip joints. If they are tight they will restrict the free swinging back of the thigh and leg when walking and running. This will tend to give a twisting motion to the pelvis and thus the back.

Test for adductor tightness   This is not easy to do yourself. The ability to stand with the knees straight and the feet wide apart will be restricted. While you are in the position for testing your iliopsoas and rectus femoris muscles ask someone to push the knee of the free hanging leg outwards. If the adductors are free it should be possible to push the thigh outwards for about ten to fifteen degrees. When they are tight they are responsible for a sense of restriction in the groin when taking a long stride forwards.

Adductor muscle stretch   Kneel on one knee, keeping the trunk straight up. Slide the other leg, with the knee kept straight, out sideways until there is a sense of tightness in that groin (see Fig. 60). Then, keeping perfectly still, push down hard with the inside of the outstretched foot for the usual seven seconds. Then

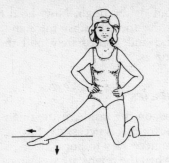

Figure 60 *The adductor muscle stretch*

relax and immediately slide the foot a little further sideways.
Repeat the usual three times and end with a final stretch.

Tensor fascia lata muscle

This is a small muscle which has a long tendon running down
the outside of the thigh. It arises from the outside rim of the
pelvis and is inserted into the outside of the knee. Its main action
is to pull the thigh outwards. It also may become tight with
prolonged sitting, especially with the legs apart. Although it is
not a major muscle it may interfere with a smooth rhythm of
walking and running if it is tight.

Tensor fascia lata test   Stand sideways to a convenient wall.
Rest the nearest outstretched hand against the wall. Cross the
leg furthest away from the wall in front of the other (see Fig.
61). Allow the hips to cave in towards the wall. To do this it is
necessary to allow the front knee to bend and also the elbow
of the arm resting against the wall. If the muscle is tight little
side bend will be possible.

  This muscle may also be tested at the same time as the iliopsoas and rectus femoris muscles: if the muscle is tight the free
leg hanging over the end of the couch will naturally tend to be
pulled sideways. Also, if the tendon is tight it will be seen and
felt as a tight groove on the outside of the thigh.

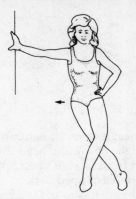

Figure 61 *Tensor fascia lata muscle stretch*

Tensor fascia lata stretch It is difficult to stretch this muscle by using a hold-relax technique so a slow stretch has to be applied. Take up the same position as for testing the muscle (Fig. 61): sideways on to a wall with the outside leg crossed in front of the other. Move the straight back leg further away from the wall, as far as it will go without undue discomfort. By bending the forward knee and the elbow of the arm resting against the wall it is possible to cave the hips in towards the wall. This will impose a stretch on the muscle. For a slow stretch this position needs to be held for about ten to fifteen seconds and to be repeated about ten times.

Chest (Thoracic) Spine: the long body stretch

If there is some wear and tear in the chest spine, you will be aware of discomfort in the middle of the chest part of the spine after sitting at a desk for some time (bent over a typewriter, for example). A simple way to counter this is to do a long body stretch exercise.

Assume the position which could best be described as that of abject submission: get down on the floor on your hands and knees. Keeping the thighs vertical at all times, slide the hands forward and bring the forehead down to rest on the ground (see

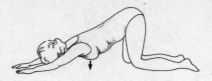

Figure 62 *The long body stretch*

Fig. 62). If you spreadeagle your straight arms to about forty-five degrees from straight above the head this will also stretch the pectoral muscles in front of your chest. Often, these also get tight after sitting over a flat-topped desk.

From this position the trick is to try and push the chest down on to the ground, and to hold this position for about ten seconds at a time, repeating ten times, with a short interval between each stretch.

This exercise is also an effective way to apply a relaxing backward stretch to the low back.

Neck exercises

The two most useful neck exercises have already (pages 148 and 150–151) been described.

Pectoral muscles

As I have just mentioned, the pectoral muscles in front of the chest also tend to get short and tight in those with sendentary occupations, giving a round-shouldered look.

The main pectoral muscles arise from the ribs close to the breast bone (sternum), and are inserted into the front of the upper part of the upper arm bone (humerus). When they are short and tight they have the effect of pulling our shoulders forward, making us look round-shouldered.

To test your own pectoral muscles, stand facing an open doorway. Stretch out both arms to about forty-five degrees from the vertical, resting the hands against each side of the doorway (see Fig. 63). Keeping the arms straight it should be possible to

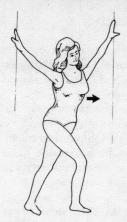

Figure 63 *Pectoral muscle stretch*

move forwards until the outstretched arms and the trunk are in the same sideways plane.

Pectoral stretch   These muscles will be stretched when doing the long body stretch, but it is not always convenient to get down on one's hands and knees.

Take up the same position as for testing the muscle, with the arms outstretched to forty-five degrees from the vertical. Move the trunk forward until these muscles feel tight. Hold this position and push hard with the hands against the sides of the doorway for the usual seven seconds. Relax and immediately move the trunk forward till the muscle again feels tight. Repeat three times, as for other hold-relax exercises.

There are other muscle groups which may become shortened and tight. Particularly if they harbour 'hot' trigger points, you will need to stretch them out and keep them stretched. To do this will require expert guidance.

Summary on excercises

There are many different exercise programmes recommended by various experts. It would seem that exercise programmes are like beer: there is no bad beer, but some brands are better than others.

I have tried to cut a way through the jungle, to explain exactly what the excercises are aiming to achieve, to give good reasons for using those which I have described, and to warn against some others that may be harmful.

You may say: what about mobility exercises? If I do not put my joints through their full range of movement will they not stiffen up?

Let's remember that our range of movement is limited by the movement allowed by our muscles. This is short of the range possible within the joints themselves. If tight muscles are relaxed the range of the joints will automatically increase to their full potential, that which is allowed by the presence of any previous wear and tear. There is only so much running in an old horse. This increased range should be maintained by everyday activities.

So, in fact, all exercise programmes are good (but see the warnings on pages 163 and 172). The act of exercising is the essential common denominator. Whatever exercises you do it is very important to stop if they hurt. The concept of having to suffer pain in order to get better has no foundation in fact. Creating pain just creates more reflex muscle tightness.

It should be realized that the act of stretching tight muscles does *not* alter the intrinsic muscle length. This is determined by the non-contractile part of the muscle: the supporting sheath round the muscle fibres and the tendons at each end. To alter the intrinsic muscle length would take months of hard work, and though such stretching may be of value to gymnasts, ballet dancers, and the like, it is of doubtful value to the rest of us.

What you *are* doing is reflexly relaxing muscle which is too tight because of increased activity in the nerves supplying the muscle fibres and muscle spindles. Obviously, the muscles will quickly tighten again after being stretched. To start with, the stretch exercises need to be repeated four to six times a day. When the muscles become more relaxed they do not tighten up again so quickly and the stretch can be maintained by twice daily stretches.

Here comes the rub. How many of us are prepared to perform a twice-daily routine of muscle stretches day in and day out to the end of our days? Very few. As with dieting, most of us eventually give up exercise routines sooner or later. Time dulls the memory of the agonies we suffered from our neck or back.

But if we carry on as we did before we got into trouble with our neck or back it is likely we shall have further trouble. 'Yes! But if I have further trouble all I need do is go back and have my back manipulated again, or acupunctured, and I shall be cured again.' Maybe, but also maybe not.

There is a built-in danger of being the passive recipient of some active treatment: 'There you are, you are cured. I have cured you. Off you go. Keep on keeping on. If you have further trouble I shall be here to treat you.' Good for business.

The best insurance against further trouble is to get the muscles more relaxed, in better tone, and those capable of protecting our spines, stronger. This means altering our way of life to include more exercise in general.

So, you start by defining which of your postural muscles are tight and by stretching them. Do not waste time stretching those which are not tight. To start with, avoid strengthening exercises. These tend to tighten up other postural muscles which may need relaxing too. Once the tight muscles are stretched out, you can think of strengthening exercises. The main muscles requiring strengthening are those which are capable of taking the strain off the spine when we bend with our knees and hips in order to lift. These are the abdominals, the rump muscles, and the main muscle mass in front of our thighs (the quadriceps) – the muscles which go floppy when we sit for long. As a general rule specific strengthening exercises for these muscles are not necessary if we increase the amount of exercise in general. Most forms of general exercise will do the required strengthening for you.

Exercising

You have had an attack of back pain. You have got the message. You need to get on the move and get fit. Some advice on how to get this increased exercise may be of help.

Walking

Most of us do little regular walking nowadays, and yet it is probably the best general exercise of all.

After an attack of back pain walking should be encouraged as soon as it is possible without undue discomfort. The distance walked should be gradually, very gradually, increased day by day. Any other more vigorous exercise should not be started before a three mile walk is possible without undue discomfort. Tight postural muscles capable of restricting the free swing of the thighs and legs should be stretched out just before setting out on a walk. Once walking for some distance has become a regular habit, the walking itself will keep them stretched out. The problem with walking is the time factor. To maintain a reasonable level of fitness it is necessary to walk for about an hour and twenty minutes, at least three times a week, so alternatives to walking may be sought.

Swimming

Swimming is an excellent way to exercise. The main problems may be access to a suitable swimming pool all the year round, and the fact that you need to be a competent swimmer to enjoy it. The water needs to be warm enough: sudden immersion in very cold water will provoke too much muscle spasm. Swimming is a completely non-weight-bearing exercise; this is its main advantage. It cannot harm our spinal joints.

Some back pain sufferers find it too uncomfortable. This is because the low back is held in the lordotic (sway-back) position when using most swimming strokes, particularly breaststroke and the like. If the discs are narrowed and the facet joints worn such a position may stress the joints and provoke painful muscle spasm. Stretching the iliopsoas and rectus femoris muscles immediately before swimming may help to solve this problem. People with neck problems have to take care for the same reasons: the breaststroke and similar styles involve a lot of neck extension which may cause pain.

The usual advice is to swim up and down the pool until you run out of steam. With improved fitness the distance covered will gradually increase.

The main problem with swimming, and with other forms of regular exercise, is boredom. This is difficult to overcome and has to be accepted. The end justifies the means. The ideal would be for exercise to be part of an enjoyable game. Unfortunately, a lot of games involving vigorous exercise have their own built-in hazards for neck and back pain sufferers.

Cycling

This is another excellent way to exercise. Unfortunately, a lot of our roads are not designed for the safe transit of cyclists, and there is, at times, a real risk of being knocked over. Then too, cycling on heavily-used roads can lead to the inhalation of toxic fumes from passing vehicles.

The modern ten-speed cycle is a bit of a hazard for back-pain sufferers: the handlebars are too low. This may involve too much bending forward of the low back. Many racing cyclists complain their backs become sore after covering some distance. If you watch them side on the reason becomes obvious: to position themselves over the pedals in order to give maximum drive to their legs, and to reduce wind resistance to a minimum, they have to bend their backs so much that they become bowed. This puts all the ligaments behind the pivot point on the stretch. With prolonged stretching they become distorted, stimulating the pain nerve endings and provoking reflex painful muscle spasm. The excessive bending in the low back could be reduced if the pelvis was rotated forwards but this is impossible because of associated tight hamstring muscles.

If you wish to cycle reverse the handlebars. Better still, change your cycle to one of the old fashioned sit-up-and-beg models.

You may not travel so fast, but you can enjoy the passing scenery, and you may arrive pain free.

If you have tight hamstrings stretch them out before cycling.

Jogging

The current popularity of jogging reflects our instinctively felt need for vigorous exercise. It is a very good way to obtain adequate exercise but it does create problems: the repetitive heel strike on a hard surface jars the spine. If the spinal joints are worn this may overstimulate the stress sensing nerves in the capsules of the facet joints, particularly if the discs have already lost some of their resilience and ability to absorb shock. This may provoke painful muscle spasm.

It has been suggested that this repetitive impact stress on the spine may accelerate the ageing process. Repetitive impact stress on the discs is known to cause this, but in the experiments which showed this the stress imposed was far greater than that which occurs while jogging. In fact, the repetitive movement is more likely to do good than harm.

If you wish to start jogging after recovery from an attack of back pain you should first walk. By the time you can walk three miles without discomfort it is reasonable to start jogging. Use well padded shoes and keep off hard surfaces as much as possible – start on grass. A twenty-minute jog at least three times a week is sufficient to maintain adequate overall fitness. If your back is sore after running some distance this may mean you have specific tight postural muscles. These need to be checked out in the way described. If you have tight muscle groups it is wise to stretch them out immediately before jogging. If you have no obvious tight muscle groups and if appropriate stretching does not relieve the pain experienced while running it is then time to call it a day. The amount of wear and tear in the spine is such that painful muscle spasm will continue to occur whenever you run.

There is one other problem particularly associated with jogging. This is known as the 'jogger's high'. After suffering considerable discomfort for some time, which is evident on the faces of those jogging, there comes a feeling of wellbeing. You feel you could go on forever.

What happens is this: the prolonged discomfort stimulates the body to produce its own painkillers, the endorphins (and other substances) which have already been described. These are responsible for the feeling of relaxed wellbeing after vigorous exercise. They have similar properties to the drug morphine — we may become addicted to them. Some runners do. People who habitually run long distances usually experience withdrawal symptoms when they have to stop running for some time: they become irritable, restless, bad tempered, sleep badly, and so on. Production of these endorphins may mask pain which may be coming from any part of our anatomy, thus blocking the body's natural warning system. We may mask any damage which is being done. As with all pleasurable addictions, in time more and more stimulus is required to produce the desired high. We have to run further and further until there is a real risk of doing permanent damage to some of our moving parts. This is a trap for the unwary jogger.

Rebound exercising

Rebound exercising is an alternative to jogging which has all of its advantages, none of its disadvantages, and some advantages all of its own.

First it should be known the author has no financial interests in the manufacture, distribution, or sale of rebound exercisers. I only wish I had.

In essence, a rebound exerciser is a circular mini-trampoline, just over a metre (3 feet) in diameter and 22.5 cm (9 inches) high. (See Fig. 64.) It consists of a firm central mat and a narrow outer rim of springs. These springs allow the central mat to give when running or jumping on the surface. It dissipates the impact stress experienced when running or jumping on a hard surface. It has one other attribute: when jumping or running the surface gives way in all directions. This gives optimum stimulation to the body's balancing mechanisms — it improves balance and co-ordination.

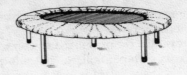

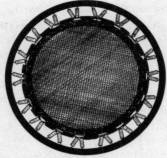

Figure 64 *A rebound exerciser*

If you have a neck or back problem it is important to use it correctly. As with jogging it is important to ensure that walking some distance is possible before starting rebounding. The main potential hazard is the imposition of repetitive impact stresses on worn facet joints, which may provoke reflex painful muscle spasm. This means neither the neck or low back should be in the sway (lordotic) position while rebounding. The neck should be held in the chin tuck-in position looking down towards the feet. The low back needs to be held so the tail is tucked in and the weight carried in front of the centre of gravity. To do this it is necessary to jog quietly on the spot, bringing the knees up in front and not kicking the heels up behind. It is wise to ensure the back and iliopsoas muscles are well stretched out immediately before rebounding (see the exercises on pages 130 and 175–6).

Rebounding is a deceptively vigorous form of exercise. Three minutes at a time is quite long enough for starters. This should be repeated three or four times a day. The length of time spent on the rebounder should be increased very gradually, not more than an extra minute each week.

After recovery from an attack of neck or back pain it is wise to stick to simple jogging on the spot before trying other exercises; until you can jog comfortably for about ten minutes. At all costs avoid high jumping. Maintaining the necessary balance to do this may easily provoke sudden contraction in the back muscles.

Rebounding is an excellent way to tighten up and strengthen the abdominal and rump muscles. No other strengthening exercises are necessary.

The problem with rebounding, as with other forms of vigorous exercise, is boredom. You do not get changes of scenery as you do with jogging. Then again, if facial expressions are anything to go by, the jogger does not much enjoy the passing scenery.

This boredom may be overcome by playing a favourite record, keeping time to the music.

Rebounding has another advantage over jogging: it can be done in the privacy of your own home, in all weathers. You need not expose yourself to the real or imagined ridicule of passers-by. If you are interested in rebounding further information is available in: *Fitness for all ages*, by James W. Fisk (Charles C. Thomas, 2600 South First Street, Springfield, Illinois 62717, USA).

Organized sport

Younger patients, just recovering from an attack of neck or back pain, often eagerly ask their doctors, 'Is it OK for me to start playing soccer [rugby, or whatever] again?' The answer to this is a qualified yes. The advantages gained from overall fitness and vigorous exercise have to be balanced against the potential hazards of each individual sport. For example, if you play soccer and you have some wear and tear in the joints at the top of the neck frequent heading of the ball will more than likely provoke a nasty headache. If this keeps happening it is time to stop. If you have marked wear and tear in your low thoracic spine due to previous Scheuermann's Disease and you notice that each time you play in the scrum in a game of rugby, your back becomes painful, then it is time to change your position in the team or change your sport.

It needs to be understood that if pain is provoked it does not necessarily mean that more damage is being done to the spine. It just means that painful muscle spasm has been provoked.

Wear and tear in the low thoracic spine is common in the young. This region of the spine is very vulnerable to stress in all sports involving a repetitive twist, such as racquet sports. If pain continues to be provoked when taking part in these sports, unless one is prepared to put up with such discomfort, they have to be stopped.

The low back is relatively well protected from twisting stresses as long as it is kept upright. Golfers are more likely to strain their low backs when picking the ball out of the hole. If pain is provoked by swinging a golf club this means the low thoracic spine is being overstressed. Shortening the golf swing may help to reduce this.

It should be restated: vigorous activities within socially-acceptable limits are unlikely to damage the spine further, but if the spine is already worn such activities may hurt. If you are prepared to put up with such hurt by all means carry on. No harmful effects will result. If not, stop the activity. If you have tight postural muscles these should always be stretched out immediately before any game.

Useful tips for everyday living

All my advice is based on the following principles:

1   Minimizing stress on the back wall of the disc which may be weakened by previous wear and tear.

2   Minimizing stress on the ligaments behind the pivot point of movement, and also on the casing of the facet joints.

3   Avoidance of excessive weight-bearing by possibly worn facet joints.

4   Avoidance of moderate prolonged stretching of ligaments, which may lead to their distortion.

5   Avoidance of prolonged muscle overuse.

First and foremost, this means correct bending and lifting. This requires full use of the hips and knees and minimum use of the back. The back should be slightly bent forward while lifting, otherwise the facet joints may be asked to carry excessive weight. All trunk twisting should be avoided whilst lifting.

When the discs are young and healthy, apart from accidents, it does not matter how you bend and lift – you are unlikely to do any harm. But if the discs are worn correct lifting becomes very important. Unfortunately by the time this happens bad habits of lifting may have become ingrained into the brain computer, and they are very difficult to change. Correct techniques of lifting should be taught at home and at school.

If you are doing something and your neck or back becomes sore, you are doing it for too long and in such a way as to provoke painful muscle spasm. It should be possible for each individual to work out ways of doing things which do not lead to pain.

Standing

Prolonged standing with a marked sway in the low back may provoke discomfort in some.

Find a small box to put one foot on. Keep changing the foot which is resting on the box. Opening the bottom cupboard under the sink and resting one foot on a shelf may make working at the sink less painful.

If a sink or bench is too low it means too much continuous bending forward in front of the centre of gravity. The neck and back muscles become fatigued and painful. If possible, the sink and ironing board height will need to be altered.

Sitting

By now you will have gathered that any prolonged sitting, however comfortable you are, is not a good thing. Make sure you have adequate low back support. Some form of padding placed at the small of the back may help some people, but not all. A rocking chair is ideal for relaxed evening sitting.

Sitting working over a flat-topped desk is potentially stressful to necks and upper backs. It may be possible to arrange a sloping working surface, such as a book rest, to allow the head to be held more upright.

Long car journeys are uncomfortable for most people with worn back joints, however well the car seat is designed. The quest for decreased wind resistance and thus improved performance has led to the lowering in the height of the modern car. This has made it impossible to design a so-called ideal seat for drivers and passengers. Reaching for the foot controls causes too much extension of the hips and knees which may cause the hamstrings to pull the pelvis round. This flexes the low back which may leave it inadequately supported. If one sits forward to counter this the knees become jammed under the dashboard or steering wheel. If the seat is inclined further backwards to counter the pull on the hamstrings then the neck has to be bent too far forwards. This, combined with the tensions involved in coping with modern day traffic, may lead to a very sore neck. Also, the average arm rests are usually inadequate and at the wrong height.

A compromise has to be reached. Get the journey over as quickly as possible, and/or have frequent breaks when you get out of the car, jump up and down and have a good stretch. Push the seat forward as far as is comfortably possible. If necessary, an extension to the foot pedals may be fitted. A small cushion in the small of the back may help some. A light sorbo-rubber collar may be a boon to sore neck sufferers, particularly passengers.

Work in the home

Various tasks around the house may be stressful to worn necks and backs. Working at the sink and ironing board have already been mentioned. Vacuuming may cause a sore back; rarely is the rigid connecting tube long enough to allow a comfortable upright stance. Holding the cord behind your back with one hand and conciously arching the back, keeping one foot well in front of the other, will help.

Getting something out of a low oven or cupboard is potentially stressful. Any twist in the back has to be avoided. Wherever possible kneel down on one knee. An eye-level oven may be a boon: you can get a squirt of fat in your eye without the need for any bending.

Putting things in and taking them out of cars and the average car boot is potentially hazardous. Lift with both hands where possible and keep any objects as close to the body as is possible. Any twisting must be avoided. Kneel when possible, or rest one or both knees against some part of the car.

Making beds can be a risky business. Kneeling down while tucking in the sheets and blankets will protect your back.

Young babies are a hazard. The muscles, particularly the abdominals, are not in very good shape after pregnancy and childbirth. Care should be taken when bending over the cot, bath, and when changing nappies. Kneel where possible. You should be able to work out how to do these things yourself so that minimum stress is imposed on the neck and back. The main thing is to try and think before you act.

Manual work

Research has shown that manual workers are no more prone to attacks of back pain than those in sedentary jobs, but obviously they need to be fitter and thus take longer to get over each attack before returning to work.

In any job involving repetitive bending and lifting the spine and muscles adjust to the habitual pattern. The danger lies in the sudden unexpected strain, or a change of job which involves the use of a different set of muscles and a different posture. Work-related back and neck injuries should be avoidable if each appointed task is carefully analyzed and appropriate steps are taken to reduce potential hazards. This is the responsibility of industrial medical officers and the like.

Gardening is considered as leisure by some but as work by others. It is foolish to expect the spine and muscles will not complain if a whole day is spent digging when it is a year since the last bout of such activity.

Make sure the tool handles are long enough, so that too much prolonged stooping is avoided. Do not stoop over for too long at a time: your ligaments may become overstretched with prolonged moderate stretching. Ten minutes at a time is probably long enough. Stand up frequently and stretch and fully arch your spine. Kneel wherever possible. A kneeling pad is helpful.

Whatever the activity it is important, as we get older, to do it regularly. Great care has to be taken after a long lay-off or in taking up a new activity.

Possible Dangers of Self Help

If you are normally fit and healthy, not too advanced in years, and you suddenly strain your neck or back, then you have joined the unhappy throng of millions of similar sufferers who have overstressed their worn spinal joints. It is extremely unlikely the resulting pain has a more serious significance.

Rarely, a growth in the spine or a spread of a growth from elsewhere may cause neck or back pain. If this has happened you are unlikely to feel otherwise fit and well. A characteristic of such a pain is its severity, particularly during the night.

Rarely, very rarely, some so-called metabolic diseases may cause alterations in the spine which may be painful.

There is a disease which mainly affects the spine, called ankylosing spondylitis. This may first present as a low back pain. It is more common in the young male.

In none of these situations will a few days rest and any local home treatment have any significant effect on the pain. But, nothing will have been lost by waiting a few days before further help is sought.

Very occasionally, some serious disease in the insides may cause a back pain, such as an eroding ulcer on the back wall of the stomach, or something which may go wrong with the prostate gland. If this happens there are most likely other symptoms present, such as long-standing indigestion, or difficulties with the waterworks.

Gynaecological problems may present with back pain. Then again, one well know gynaecologist has stated that as a general rule back pain comes from the back.

Very rarely (I have seen three cases in the past thirty-odd years of practice) there is a massive rupture of a disc in the low back which may press on the nerve roots inside the spinal canal.

If nothing is done about this quickly there may be permanent damage to the nerves.

This usually happens very quickly. There is a sudden severe back pain which quickly tends to spread down both legs, which may feel weak. The danger signs are a feeling of numbness in the area which would be in contact with a saddle, if you have ever sat on one. There may be problems with the waterworks – difficulty in passing urine and some loss of control. Also, if you are male and game enough to try, you may find you are impotent.

If any or all of these symptoms are present urgent surgical help is required, preferably in a matter of a few hours. The longer such surgical relief is left the more likely is some permanent nerve damage.

If you have reached this far I offer my thanks and congratulations. If you have read and understood what has been written I have achieved my purpose.

Neck and back pain need not and should not become an ongoing problem, making life a constant misery. Loss of compliance in our joints, which goes with ageing, should not hurt. With increasing age, and hopefully good sense, we should learn not to put excessive stress on our worn joints.

Understanding the problem is half the battle. The other half is having the will to do something about it: keeping fit and active, in a non-stressful way, and learning to recognize when our coping systems are becoming overloaded.

Index

stretching exercises, 127
tension headaches, 144–6,
152–3, Fig. 49
trapezius muscle, 150
treatment, 95–7
whiplash injuries, 155
tuberculosis, 115

ulcers, stomach, 195
upper trapezius stretch exercise,
150–1
urination, 195, 196

vertebrae: ageing process, 79
in chest, 32–3
fractures, 101
in neck, 30–2, Figs. 16, 17
Scheuermann's Disease, 80–5,
Fig. 35
structure and function, 16–19,
Figs. 2, 3

visco-elasticity, 20, 35

wakefulness, 62
walking, 167, 169, 184
water beds, 108
well-being: jogger's high, 187
manipulation, 126–7
whiplash injury, 100–2, 103,
154–5
women: cervical spondylosis, 79
gynaecological problems, 195
overloaded coping system
syndrome, 104–5
work: in the home, 192–3
manual, 82–3, 193–4
wry neck, 69, 155–6

X-rays, 78, 79, 82–3, 101, 135,
154

yoga, 158